The Great American EAT-RIGHT Cookbook

140 Great-Tasting, Good-for-You Recipes

JEANNE BESSER
COLLEEN DOYLE, MS, RD

PHOTOGRAPHY BY HOLLY SASNETT

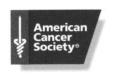

American Cancer Society®

Published by
American Cancer Society
250 Williams Street NW
Atlanta, GA 30303-1002 USA

5 4 3 2 1   07 08 09 10 11

Library of Congress Cataloging-in-Publication Data

Besser, Jeanne.
 The great American eat-right cookbook / Jeanne Besser and Colleen Doyle.
     p. cm.
 ISBN-13: 978-0-944235-93-5 (hardcover)
 ISBN-10: 0-944235-93-X (hardcover)
 1. Quick and easy cookery. 2. Low-fat diet—Recipes. 3. Low-calorie
diet—Recipes. I. Doyle, Colleen. II. Title.

 TX833.5.B4877155 2007
 641.5'55—dc22

                              2007021930

Printed in the United States of America

PHOTOGRAPHY: Holly Sasnett, Atlanta, GA
COVER PHOTOGRAPH: Holly Sasnett, Atlanta, GA
FOOD STYLING: Jeanne Besser, Atlanta, GA
NUTRITIONAL ANALYSIS: Madelyn L. Wheeler, MS, RD, Zionsville, IN
DESIGN: Jill Dible, Atlanta, GA

AMERICAN CANCER SOCIETY
EDITOR: Jill Russell
MANAGING EDITOR: Rebecca Teaff
BOOK PUBLISHING MANAGER: Candace Magee
DIRECTOR, BOOK PUBLISHING: Len Boswell
STRATEGIC DIRECTOR, CONTENT: Chuck Westbrook

Quantity discounts on bulk purchases of this book are available. Book excerpts can also be created to fit specific needs. For information, please contact the American Cancer Society, Health Promotions Publishing, 250 Williams Street NW, Atlanta, GA 30303-1002, or send an e-mail to trade.sales@cancer.org.

For more information about cancer, contact your American Cancer Society at **1-800-ACS-2345** or www.cancer.org.

COVER: *Poached Salmon With Mango Salsa*. For recipe, see page 40.

BACK COVER: *Oven–Baked Potato Chips* and *"Deconstructed" Apple Crisp*.
For recipes, see pages 104 and 172.

ABOUT THE NUTRITION INFORMATION: The nutrition information shown for each recipe represents one serving. Optional ingredients and ingredients listed without measurement (such as salt and pepper, unless a specific measurement is given) are not represented in the analysis. When two choices are given, the first was used in the analysis.

CONTENTS

Recipe List iv
Introduction vi

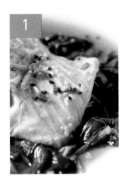

MAIN
COURSES

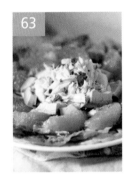

SOUPS,
SALADS, AND
SANDWICHES

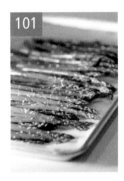

SIDES

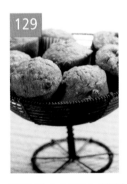

BREAKFAST

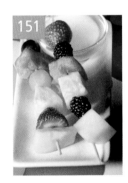

SNACKS

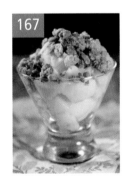

DESSERTS

How to Stock Your Kitchen to Promote Healthy Eating 188
Recipe Makeovers 101: Three Steps to Healthier Meals 190
American Cancer Society Guidelines on Nutrition and Physical Activity 191
Index 192

RECIPE LIST

MAIN COURSES

Broccoli, Garlic, and Lemon Penne 3
Grilled Chicken Breasts with Pineapple Salsa 4
Wasabi Salmon Burgers 5
Provençal Fish 6
Oven-Roasted Herbed Turkey Breast 7
Southern Shrimp and Sausage 9
Tofu Stir-Fry with Peanut Sauce 10
Shrimp and Asparagus Risotto 11
Grilled Baja–Style Fish Tacos 13
Microwave Thai Red Curry Salmon 14
Ginger-Poached Salmon with Orange and Honey 15
Mussels with Fennel, Leek, and Grape Tomatoes 16
Tomato–Fennel Tofu Bake 18
Tandoori-Style Chicken 19
Portobellos Stuffed with Spinach, Brown Rice, and Feta . . . 21
Olé Pasta Casserole 22
Tasty Turkey Tacos 23
Green Curry Shrimp 24
Lower-Fat Mac-n-Cheese 26
Apricot–Orange Baked Chicken 27
Crunchy "Oven-Fried" Chicken Nuggets 28
Steamed Pesto-Rolled Tilapia with Vegetables 29
Pork Tenderloin Topped with Fall Fruits 31
Chicken Chili 32
Chicken and Barley Stew 33
Homemade Pizza 35
Whole Wheat Penne with Roasted Vegetable Sauce 36
Chicken and Broccoli Stir-Fry 37
Grilled Teriyaki Chicken Kebabs 38
Quick Chicken Cacciatore 39
Poached Salmon with Mango Salsa 40
Moroccan Spiced Chicken with Vegetable Couscous 42
Black Bean and Butternut Squash Chili 43
Skillet Tilapia with Sautéed Spinach 45
Mini Meatloaves 46
Savory Salmon and Leek Packets 47
Shrimp, Bean, and Feta Bake 48
Ratatouille with Beans 49
Salmon in Asian Broth 50
Fig, Ginger, and Butternut Squash Risotto 52
Mexican "Lasagna" 53
Moo Shu Chicken Lettuce Wraps 55
Fettuccine with Tomato–Herb Sauce 56
Stir-Fried Pork, Green Beans, and Shiitake Mushrooms . . . 57
Stuffed Greek Chicken Breasts 58
Seafood Stew 60

SOUPS, SALADS, AND SANDWICHES

Southwest Chicken Tortilla Soup 64
Aromatic Butternut Squash and Apple Soup 65
Black Bean Soup with Cilantro Cream 66
Super Veggie Soup 67
Chicken and White Bean Soup 69
Red Clam Chowder 70
Mushroom–Barley Soup 71
Lentil–Vegetable Soup 72
Roasted Root Vegetable Soup 73
Tuna Melt 74
Barbecue Chicken Quesadilla 75
Crab Salad with Grapefruit, Avocado, and Baby Greens . . . 76
Eggs-traordinary Taco 78
Curried Chicken Salad 79
Spicy Soba Salad 80
Mediterranean Chicken Salad 81
Asian Beef Salad 83
Tomatoes Stuffed with Shrimp Salad 84
Tuna–Bean Salad 85
Turkey Burgers with Cranberry Chutney 86
Greek Chicken and Tzatziki Pitas 87
Southwestern Bean Burgers 88
Lamb Burgers with Tomato–Olive Relish 89
Shrimp, Watermelon, and Avocado Salad 91
Turkey Roll-up 92
Quinoa and Corn Salad with Rosemary 93
Quesadilla with Beans, Corn, and Green Chiles 94

Spinach, Portobello, and Roasted Red Pepper Salad 95
Beet, Orange, and Arugula Salad 96
Roast Beef Roll-Up 97
Wheat Berry Salad with Almonds and Dried Cherries 98

SIDES

Chunky Vegetable Salad 102
Carrot–Raisin–Apple Salad 103
Oven–Baked Potato Chips 104
Sweet Potato Fries 106
Caraway Cole Slaw 107
Garlic Mashed Potatoes 108
Arugula and Parmigiano–Reggiano Salad 109
Tabbouleh Salad 111
Greens and Herb Salad 112
Whipped Cider Sweet Potatoes 113
Black Bean and Corn Salad 115
Braised Red Cabbage and Apples 116
Sautéed Green Beans and Grape Tomatoes 117
Brown Rice Pilaf 118
Basmati Rice and Chickpea Pilaf 119
Lemon-Roasted Asparagus 120
Orange–Glazed Baby Carrots 122
Eggplant Spread 123
Roasted Potatoes and Baby Carrots 124
Sautéed Spinach with Garlic 125
Roasted Brussels Sprouts 126

BREAKFAST

Ham and Vegetable Frittata 130
Brown Sugar Yogurt Parfait 131
Raspberry–Peach Yogurt Smoothie 132
Whole Grain Gingerbread Waffles 134
Strawberry–Banana Smoothie 135
Pumpkin-Spice Pancakes 136
Buttermilk Bran Muffins 137
Tomato and Basil Frittata 139
Baked Eggs Florentine 140

Banana Pancakes 141
Carrot–Applesauce Muffins 142
Fruity Morning Oatmeal 144
Dried Fruit Compote 145
Oatmeal–Raisin Scones 147
Ginger–Cranberry Granola 148
Blueberry–Peach–Pomegranate Smoothie 149

SNACKS

Cheesy Pita Crisps 152
Rosemary Popcorn 153
Pepperoni Tortilla Pizza 155
Chili-Spiced Popcorn 156
Veggie Tortilla Pizza 157
Creamy Peanut Butter Dip 158
Mediterranean Tuna Pâté 159
Fruit Skewers with Yogurt Dipping Sauce 160
Homemade Baked Tortilla Chips 162
Fresh Tomato Salsa 163
Tomatillo Salsa 164

DESSERTS

Mint-Chocolate Meringue Cookies 169
Almond Macaroons 170
Two-Bite Brownies 171
"Deconstructed" Apple Crisp 172
Mock Berry Crème Brûlée 174
Oatmeal–Raisin Cookies 175
Chocolate Chip–Sour Cream Coffee Babycakes 177
Microwave "Baked" Apples 178
Chocolate–Cherry Frozen Yogurt 179
Strawberries with Balsamic Glaze 181
Orange–Cherry Biscotti 182
Homemade Berry Frozen Yogurt 183
Pink Grapefruit Granita 184
Chocolate–Almond Biscotti 186
Chocolate-Covered Strawberries 187

INTRODUCTION

Eating more healthfully is something many of us aspire to and something that can seem daunting. Time is at a premium, old habits can be hard to break and, frankly, everyone wants food that *tastes* good. Without a roadmap, it can be difficult to make healthy choices.

But we have good news. While eating right *can* be a challenge, with a wide variety of quick, tasty, and healthy recipes for everything from breakfasts to desserts, it doesn't have to be. Grab your mixer and pull out your measuring cups. You want to eat right, and we want to help.

Welcome to *The Great American Eat-Right Cookbook*. This collection of delicious recipes is designed to motivate, captivate, encourage, and inspire. From familiar weeknight standbys and guest-worthy entrees to quick and easy snacks and sumptuous sweets, each turn of the page offers a recipe that is sure to please. Whether you are just learning your way around the kitchen or have a bit more culinary experience, these approachable, "can-do" recipes—with helpful tips along the way—will help you turn out dishes savored by family and friends alike.

We're all busy. Hectic schedules, work, family, and the obligations of everyday life can combine to make a fast meal a necessity. Most of the recipes in the following pages can be made quickly and contain ingredients you already have in your cupboard. Keeping healthy basics on hand—canned beans, frozen fruits and vegetables, canned no-salt-added vegetables, and whole wheat pastas and flour, to name a few—can make a huge difference. See "How to Stock Your Kitchen to Promote Healthy Eating" on pages 188–189 for more help in planning ahead so you can make a great meal fast.

These recipes also pack a nutritious punch. You will discover the wonders of good-for-you recipes that include more of the things you want—fruits, vegetables, whole grains—and less of the things you don't—saturated fat, sodium, and sugar.

But let's face it: flavor matters. There are lots of ways to make dishes better for you, but if they don't taste good, it doesn't matter how healthy they are—they won't be eaten. Throughout the book, these recipes get an extra kick from fresh herbs, abundant spices, flavored vinegars, and more unusual ingredients like chili paste and chutney. The flavorful additions you'll find throughout the book, even ones you might think would be forbidden in a "healthy" diet (in moderation, of course!), make a healthy meal one worth craving.

We also give you ideas for how you can cut calories and increase nutrients, no matter what you're cooking. There are many ways to cut down on calories without sacrificing flavor. It's also easy to boost the nutrients by adding more fruits, vegetables, and whole grains to recipes. Take a look at "Recipe Makeovers 101: Three Steps to Healthier Meals," on page 190, for specific tips on making over almost any recipe.

At the bottom of each recipe, you'll find nutrition information. Use this information to make healthy, informed, and *balanced* choices throughout the day. Keep that word in mind—balance. It's okay to have a few bites of something sweet—just don't have ten bites. It's okay to have some fat in your diet, especially healthy fats. The goal should not be to deprive yourself, but to eat a healthy and well-balanced diet. And because it's important to watch *how much* you eat—and not just *what* you eat—these recipes have built-in portion control: the number of servings per recipe reflects appropriate portion sizes, making it easier for you to keep calories under control.

We all want to lower our risk of cancer, heart disease, and diabetes. Here are the most important ways to improve your health and reduce your risk for all these chronic diseases: don't smoke, watch your weight, stay active, and make healthy food choices. The "American Cancer Society Guidelines on Nutrition and Physical Activity" on page 191 provide important information on the choices everyone can make to improve their overall health.

Small steps matter. Each step you take toward better health is an important and positive one. Try to eat one cup more of fruits and vegetables each day. Choose whole grains over refined grains when possible. Limit the amount of processed and red meats you eat. Choose foods and beverages in amounts that will help you achieve and maintain a healthy weight.

Our hope is that these recipes will inspire you to get cooking, motivate you to make healthier choices, and encourage you to try something new: a new recipe, a new food, a new preparation method. We encourage you to make a commitment to yourself and make the choice to "eat right." Challenge yourself to experiment with new and different ingredients. Challenge yourself to try a new recipe each week. Challenge yourself to add your own unique twist to the recipes in these pages to make them your own. And challenge yourself each day to take a step toward better health.

The Great American Eat-Right Cookbook will introduce you to delicious—and nutritious—recipes to savor with your family and friends. Have fun, enjoy, and live well!

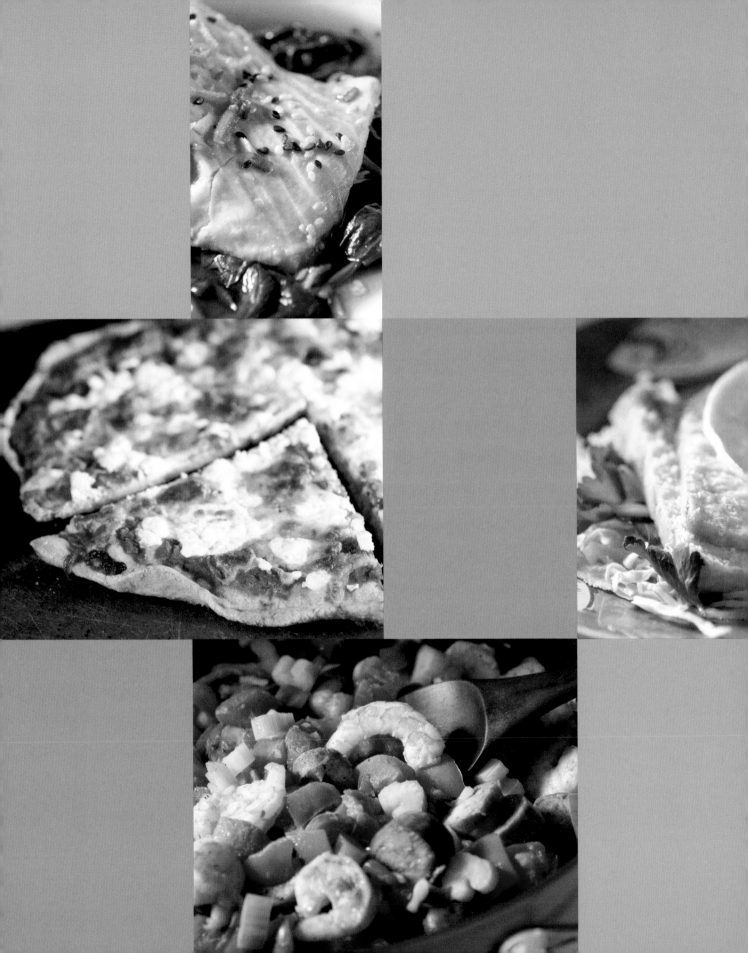

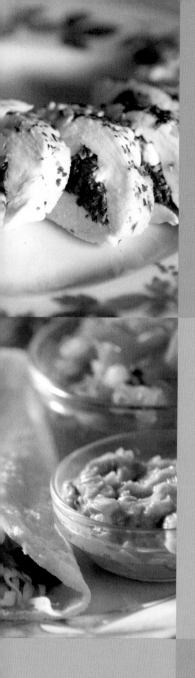

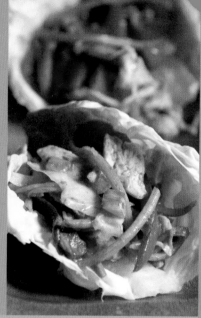

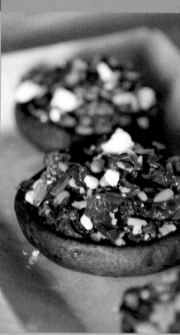

MAIN COURSES

Great for the family yet good enough for guests, these dishes are flavorful, versatile, and inspiring, and will leave family and friends alike wondering if you've spent hours slaving away in the kitchen! Whatever your culinary skills, these recipes come together quickly and will give you a great sense of satisfaction. Pick a pasta, find a new fish, try a taco. Spice up your life by adding some of these dishes to your weekly repertoire of favorites.

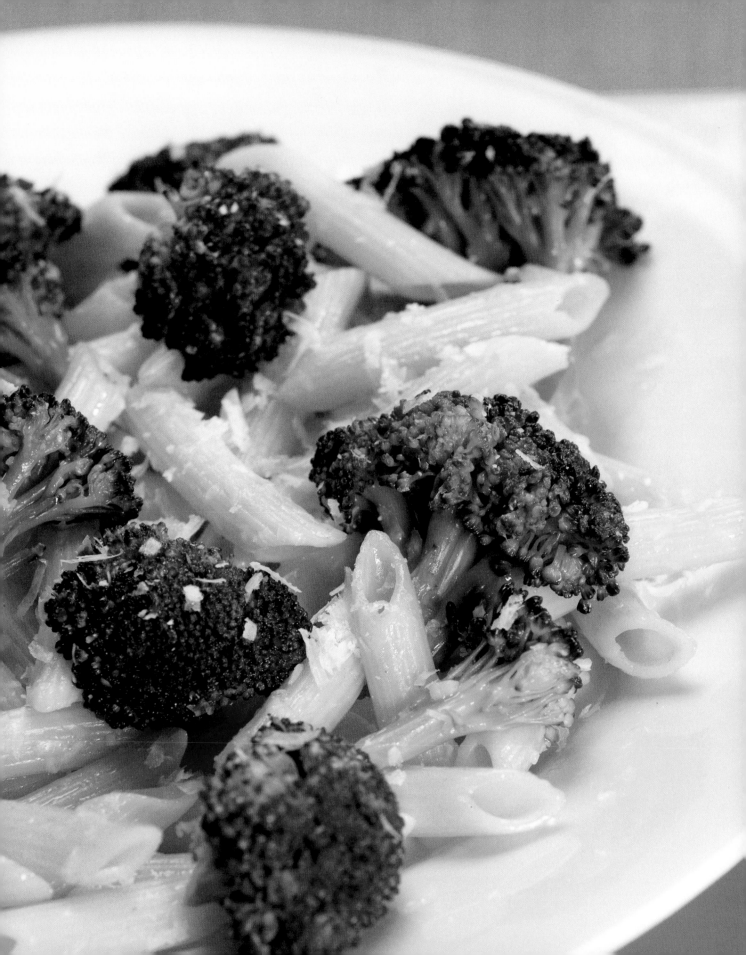

BROCCOLI, GARLIC, AND LEMON PENNE

For quicker prep, buy bagged broccoli florets. For more cheese flavor and fewer calories, grate your own Parmesan cheese with a Microplane grater, a small-holed handheld grater. It produces a finer shred, so you get more coverage with less cheese.

SERVES 4 / PREP TIME: 15 MINUTES OR LESS / TOTAL TIME: 30 MINUTES OR LESS

½ pound penne pasta
5 cups broccoli florets or 1 (12-ounce) bag broccoli florets
¼ cup extra–virgin olive oil
10 garlic cloves, thinly sliced

½ cup reduced–sodium chicken broth
Grated zest of 1 lemon
Salt and freshly ground black pepper
¼ cup freshly grated Parmesan cheese

Prepare penne according to package directions for al dente (just firm). Two to three minutes before penne is ready, add broccoli. Finish cooking, drain, and set aside.

Meanwhile, in a large skillet over medium-high heat, add oil. Sauté the garlic for 1 to 2 minutes, or until aromatic and beginning to color.

Add broth and bring to a boil for 3 to 5 minutes, or until reduced by half, stirring frequently. Add pasta, broccoli, and lemon zest and cook until coated with sauce. Season generously with salt and pepper. Transfer to serving bowl and top with cheese.

Broccoli is high in folic acid, vitamins C and K, and fiber. It's also one of the richest vegetable sources of calcium, iron, and magnesium.

Per Serving	
Calories	395
Calories from Fat	155
Total Fat	17.0 g
Saturated Fat	3.0 g
Trans Fat	0.0 g
Polyunsaturated Fat	2.0 g
Monounsaturated Fat	10.7 g
Cholesterol	5 mg
Sodium	135 mg
Total Carbohydrate	50 g
Dietary Fiber	5 g
Sugars	4 g
Protein	13 g

GRILLED CHICKEN BREASTS WITH PINEAPPLE SALSA

Grilled chicken breasts get a breath of freshness from this vibrant fruit salsa.
When it comes to making salsa, think outside the "vegetable box."
Fruit adds sweetness to counterbalance the savory ingredients.

SERVES 4 / PREP TIME: 30 MINUTES OR LESS / TOTAL TIME: 45 MINUTES OR LESS

---

2 teaspoons olive oil
2 teaspoons plus 2 tablespoons fresh
  lime juice, divided
1 pound boneless, skinless chicken
  breasts, pounded to uniform thickness
Salt and freshly ground black pepper
2 cups chopped fresh ripe pineapple

¼ cup seeded and chopped red bell
  pepper
2 tablespoons chopped fresh mint
2 tablespoons finely chopped red onion
1 small jalapeño, seeded and finely
  chopped
1 teaspoon honey

In a shallow plate, combine oil and 2 teaspoons lime juice. Add chicken, turning to coat, and marinate for 15 minutes.

Preheat a lightly oiled grill to medium-high.

Remove chicken from marinade and sprinkle with salt and pepper. Grill chicken for 5 to 8 minutes per side, or until cooked through. Remove from grill and let rest for 5 minutes before slicing.

Meanwhile, in a bowl, combine pineapple, bell pepper, mint, onion, jalapeño, honey, and the remaining 2 tablespoons lime juice.

Slice chicken and top with salsa.

Pineapple salsa can also be served with Homemade Baked Tortilla Chips (page 162) as an appetizer.

Per Serving	
Calories	250
Calories from Fat	40
Total Fat	4.5 g
Saturated Fat	1.0 g
Trans Fat	0.0 g
Polyunsaturated Fat	0.9 g
Monounsaturated Fat	2.2 g
Cholesterol	65 mg
Sodium	60 mg
Total Carbohydrate	28 g
Dietary Fiber	3 g
Sugars	23 g
Protein	25 g

WASABI SALMON BURGERS

Fresh ginger, Asian (also known as toasted) sesame oil, and soy sauce give these salmon burgers an Asian twist. Flavorful wasabi mayonnaise seals the deal! They're so good, you don't need a bun.

SERVES 4 / PREP TIME: 15 MINUTES OR LESS / TOTAL TIME: 30 MINUTES OR LESS

1 garlic clove
2 teaspoons coarsely chopped fresh ginger
1 pound salmon fillets, skin removed and cut into large pieces
1/2 cup panko bread crumbs
1/4 cup finely chopped red bell pepper
3 scallions, white and light green parts only, thinly sliced, divided

4 teaspoons reduced–sodium soy sauce, divided
1 teaspoon Asian sesame oil
1/4 cup good-quality light mayonnaise, such as Hellmann's
1 teaspoon wasabi paste, or to taste
1 teaspoon finely chopped fresh ginger

In a food processor with the motor running, add garlic and ginger and process until finely chopped. Scrape down sides and add salmon. Pulse until the salmon pieces are about 1/4-inch in size, with some smaller and larger pieces. Transfer to a bowl and stir in panko, bell pepper, 2 scallions, 2 teaspoons soy sauce, and sesame oil. Form into four patties.

Lightly coat a large skillet with nonstick cooking spray. Over medium-high heat, cook burgers for 3 to 4 minutes per side, or until cooked through and golden.

Meanwhile, in a bowl, combine mayonnaise, wasabi paste, finely chopped ginger, and the remaining 2 teaspoons soy sauce and scallion.

Top burgers with a dollop of flavored mayonnaise.

Panko, also known as Japanese bread crumbs, is coarser than standard bread crumbs. Using it in this recipe lightens the burgers. Panko is available in the Asian foods section of many supermarkets. If panko is not available, you can substitute unseasoned bread crumbs, but the texture of the burgers will be slightly different.

Per Serving
Calories 295
  Calories from Fat 145
Total Fat . . . . 16.0 g
  Saturated Fat . . . . 2.8 g
  Trans Fat . . . . 0.0 g
  Polyunsaturated Fat . . . . 5.4 g
  Monounsaturated Fat . . . . . . 6.4 g
Cholesterol . . . . 80 mg
Sodium . . . . 425 mg
Total Carbohydrate . . . . 9 g
  Dietary Fiber . . . . 1 g
  Sugars . . . . 3 g
Protein . . . . 26 g

PROVENÇAL FISH

In this dish, the fish actually cooks in a fragrant, rich tomato sauce studded with olives, capers, and herbs. Use a hearty, thick white fish fillet, such as red snapper, halibut, or cod, that can stand up to a bold topping. For added color, mix Kalamata olives with green olives.

The elegant presentation and bountiful flavors of this dish make it a great option for entertaining. Serve alongside rice or pasta to absorb every last drop of sauce.

SERVES 6 / PREP TIME: 15 MINUTES OR LESS / TOTAL TIME: 45 MINUTES OR LESS

---

1 tablespoon olive oil
1 onion, thinly sliced
3 garlic cloves, thinly sliced
1/8 teaspoon crushed red pepper flakes, optional
1 (28-ounce) can crushed tomatoes
1/2 cup sliced pimento–stuffed green olives

1/4 cup capers, drained
1/2 teaspoon dried thyme
1/2 teaspoon dried basil
1/4 teaspoon dried rosemary, crumbled
1 1/2 pounds red snapper fillets or other white fish
2 tablespoons chopped fresh Italian parsley, optional

In a large skillet over medium-high heat, add oil. Sauté the onion for 5 to 8 minutes, or until softened. Add garlic and red pepper flakes and sauté for 1 minute. Add tomatoes, olives, capers, thyme, basil, and rosemary and bring to boil. Reduce the heat and simmer for 10 minutes, stirring occasionally. Add fish and top with sauce. Cover and simmer for 8 to 10 minutes. Sprinkle with parsley.

Tomatoes and seafood are a great combo.
In addition to providing lycopene,
tomatoes are also a source of vitamin C.

Per Serving	
Calories	220
Calories from Fat	55
Total Fat	6.0 g
Saturated Fat	1.0 g
Trans Fat	0.0 g
Polyunsaturated Fat	1.0 g
Monounsaturated Fat	3.1 g
Cholesterol	40 mg
Sodium	840 mg
Total Carbohydrate	15 g
Dietary Fiber	4 g
Sugars	8 g
Protein	26 g

OVEN-ROASTED HERBED TURKEY BREAST

There's no need to wait until Thanksgiving to enjoy turkey. A turkey breast makes a great mid-week dinner. Stuffing fragrant fresh herbs under the skin infuses the meat with subtle flavorings.

Use leftovers for sandwiches, if anything remains…

SERVES 6 / PREP TIME: 15 MINUTES OR LESS / TOTAL TIME: 1 HOUR AND 30 MINUTES OR LESS

2 tablespoons finely chopped fresh Italian parsley
1 tablespoon fresh thyme leaves
1 tablespoon finely chopped fresh rosemary
1 tablespoon finely chopped shallot

2 teaspoons butter (²/₃ tablespoon), room temperature
1 (3¹/₂- to 4-pound) bone-in half turkey breast with skin, excess fat removed
Kosher or sea salt and freshly ground black pepper

Preheat the oven to 350 degrees. Lightly coat an 8-by-8-inch baking pan with nonstick cooking spray.

In a bowl, combine parsley, thyme, rosemary, shallot, and butter.

Place turkey in the baking pan. With your fingers, loosen turkey skin from the bird, taking care not to tear the skin. Spread the herb mixture between the skin and meat. Sprinkle the skin with salt and pepper.

Bake for 1 hour to 1 hour and 10 minutes, or until instant-read thermometer registers 165 degrees. Let rest for 10 minutes before slicing.

Cooking turkey or chicken with the skin on will keep the dish moist. To reduce calories and fat, remove the skin after cooking.

Per Serving
Calories 355
  Calories from Fat 135
Total Fat . . . . 15.0 g
  Saturated Fat . . . . 4.6 g
  Trans Fat . . . . 0.0 g
  Polyunsaturated Fat . . . . 3.3 g
  Monounsaturated Fat . . . . . . 4.8 g
Cholesterol . . . . 140 mg
Sodium . . . . 125 mg
Total Carbohydrate . . . . 1 g
  Dietary Fiber . . . . 0 g
  Sugars . . . . 0 g
Protein . . . . 52 g

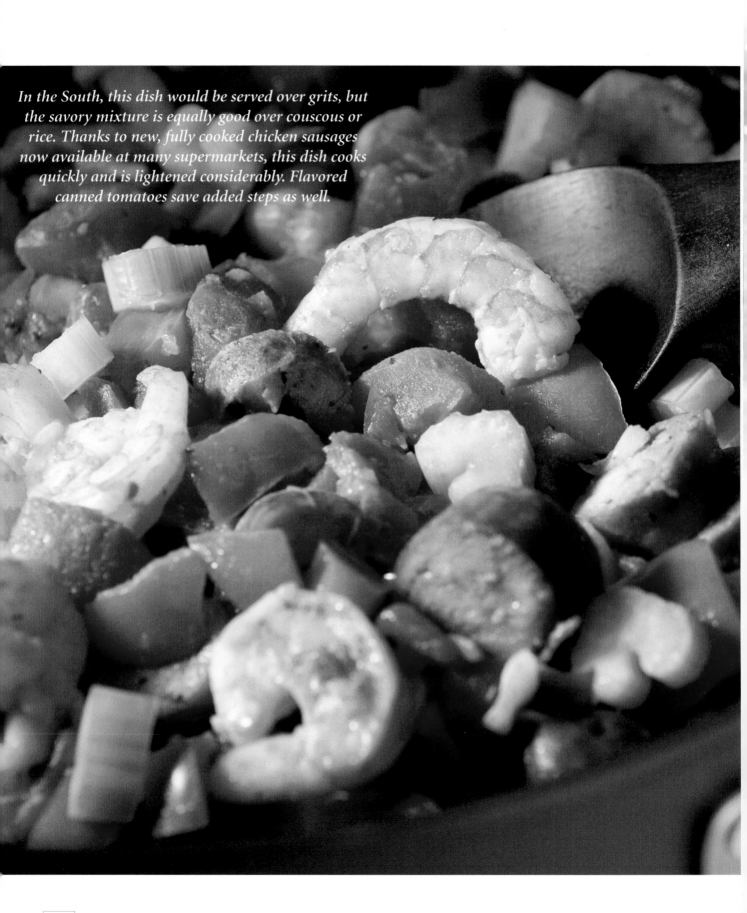

In the South, this dish would be served over grits, but the savory mixture is equally good over couscous or rice. Thanks to new, fully cooked chicken sausages now available at many supermarkets, this dish cooks quickly and is lightened considerably. Flavored canned tomatoes save added steps as well.

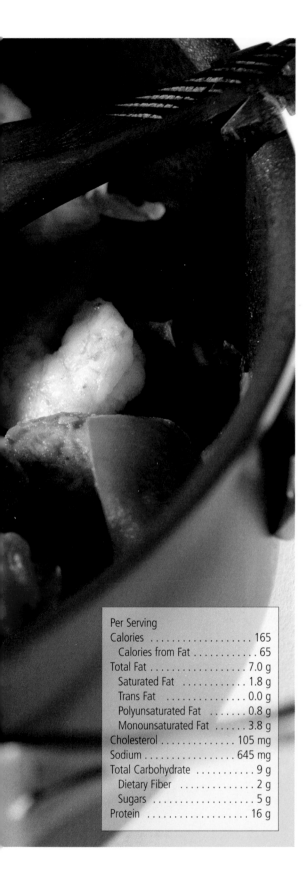

SOUTHERN SHRIMP AND SAUSAGE

SERVES 6 / PREP TIME: 15 MINUTES OR LESS / TOTAL TIME: 45 MINUTES OR LESS

1 tablespoon olive oil
1 onion, chopped
1 red bell pepper, seeded and chopped
1 green bell pepper, seeded and chopped
1 celery stalk, sliced
2 fully cooked Andouille or other flavored chicken
  sausages (half of a 12-ounce package), sliced
¼ teaspoon Creole seasoning or pinch of cayenne pepper,
  or to taste
1 (14½-ounce) can diced tomatoes with basil, garlic,
  and oregano
1 pound medium shrimp, peeled and deveined
Salt and freshly ground black pepper

In a large skillet over medium heat, add oil. Sauté the onion, both bell peppers, and celery for 5 to 8 minutes. Add sausages and Creole seasoning and sauté for 2 minutes. Add tomatoes and their juice. Reduce the heat and simmer for 5 to 10 minutes, or until thickened, stirring occasionally. Add shrimp and cook for 3 to 5 minutes, or until cooked through. Season with salt and pepper.

Per Serving	
Calories	165
Calories from Fat	65
Total Fat	7.0 g
Saturated Fat	1.8 g
Trans Fat	0.0 g
Polyunsaturated Fat	0.8 g
Monounsaturated Fat	3.8 g
Cholesterol	105 mg
Sodium	645 mg
Total Carbohydrate	9 g
Dietary Fiber	2 g
Sugars	5 g
Protein	16 g

For maximum flavor without maximum fat, use a spicy precooked chicken sausage like Aidells Organic Cajun-Style Andouille Smoked Chicken Sausage. If that brand is not available, substitute another cooked chicken sausage.

TOFU STIR-FRY WITH PEANUT SAUCE

If you've never tried tofu, this simple, flavor-packed recipe is a good place to start. Have all of your ingredients ready to go before starting to cook—and feel free to add any other vegetables you like, such as snow peas or broccoli.

Serve the finished stir-fry over steaming brown rice.

SERVES 3 / PREP TIME: 15 MINUTES OR LESS / TOTAL TIME: 30 MINUTES OR LESS

1 tablespoon peanut oil, divided
1 (14- to 16-ounce) block extra-firm tofu, drained, patted dry, and cut into 1-inch cubes
1 red bell pepper, seeded and thinly sliced
2 to 3 garlic cloves, minced
1/2-inch piece fresh ginger, peeled and finely chopped

3/4 cup frozen peas
1 bunch (4 to 6) scallions, sliced
1 tablespoon reduced–sodium soy sauce or fish sauce
1/8 teaspoon crushed red pepper flakes, or to taste
2 tablespoons peanut butter
2 tablespoons chopped fresh cilantro
Juice of 1/2 fresh lime

In a wok or large nonstick skillet over high heat, add half the oil. Add the tofu and cook without stirring for 2 minutes. Flip and cook for 2 minutes to get a light brown sear on a couple of sides of the cubes. Remove tofu from the pan and keep warm.

Add the remaining oil. Sauté bell pepper for 2 to 3 minutes, or until crisp-tender. Add garlic, ginger, peas, and scallions and sauté for 2 to 3 minutes, or until the peas are bright green. Push the vegetables to one side and add soy sauce, red pepper flakes, and peanut butter, stirring to melt the peanut butter into the soy sauce. Add tofu cubes, cilantro, and lime juice and stir to coat the vegetables and tofu with the peanut sauce.

Per Serving	
Calories	235
Calories from Fat	115
Total Fat	13.0 g
Saturated Fat	2.4 g
Trans Fat	0.0 g
Polyunsaturated Fat	4.6 g
Monounsaturated Fat	5.2 g
Cholesterol	0 mg
Sodium	355 mg
Total Carbohydrate	16 g
Dietary Fiber	5 g
Sugars	8 g
Protein	16 g

Soy products, such as tofu, are an excellent source of protein and a good alternative to red meat.

SHRIMP AND ASPARAGUS RISOTTO

*Risotto, a slow-cooking creamy rice dish made with short-grain,
highly glutinous rice, is a mainstay of Northern Italian cooking.*

*The secret to perfect risotto is the slow and gradual addition of broth. While it is not
essential to warm the broth first, it does help maintain a constant cooking temperature.*

*Use asparagus of medium thickness for more even cooking.
If using thicker spears, add them earlier; thinner spears should be added later.*

SERVES 6 / PREP TIME: 15 MINUTES OR LESS / TOTAL TIME: 45 MINUTES OR LESS

4 to 5 cups reduced–sodium chicken
broth
1 tablespoon olive oil
1½ cups Arborio or Carnaroli rice
1 cup dry white wine
1 bunch asparagus, cut into 1-inch
pieces (approximately 2 cups), tough
bottoms removed

¾ pound shrimp, peeled and deveined
¼ cup chopped fresh Italian parsley
2 tablespoons thinly sliced fresh chives
¾ cup freshly grated Parmesan cheese
Salt and freshly ground black pepper

In a saucepan, bring the chicken broth to a light simmer. Cover and keep warm over very low heat.

In a large saucepan or stockpot over medium heat, add oil. Sauté the rice for 1 minute. Add wine and stir until almost completely absorbed.

Begin slowly adding the broth, ½ cup at a time, stirring frequently. Wait until each addition is almost completely absorbed before adding more, 3 to 5 minutes for each addition. After 20 minutes, add asparagus and shrimp. Stir to combine and to prevent sticking. Continue to add broth, stirring frequently, for 8 to 10 minutes, or until the risotto has a creamy texture but is still slightly firm to the bite. You might not need to use all of the liquid.

Stir parsley, chives, and cheese into the risotto. Season with salt and pepper and serve immediately.

Use a sturdy, heavy-bottomed pan to prevent sticking and overcooking. Look for a pan with high sides, like a stockpot, to prevent moisture from evaporating too quickly.

Per Serving	
Calories	285
Calories from Fat	65
Total Fat	7.0 g
Saturated Fat	2.5 g
Trans Fat	0.0 g
Polyunsaturated Fat	0.7 g
Monounsaturated Fat	3.0 g
Cholesterol	75 mg
Sodium	505 mg
Total Carbohydrate	37 g
Dietary Fiber	1 g
Sugars	2 g
Protein	18 g

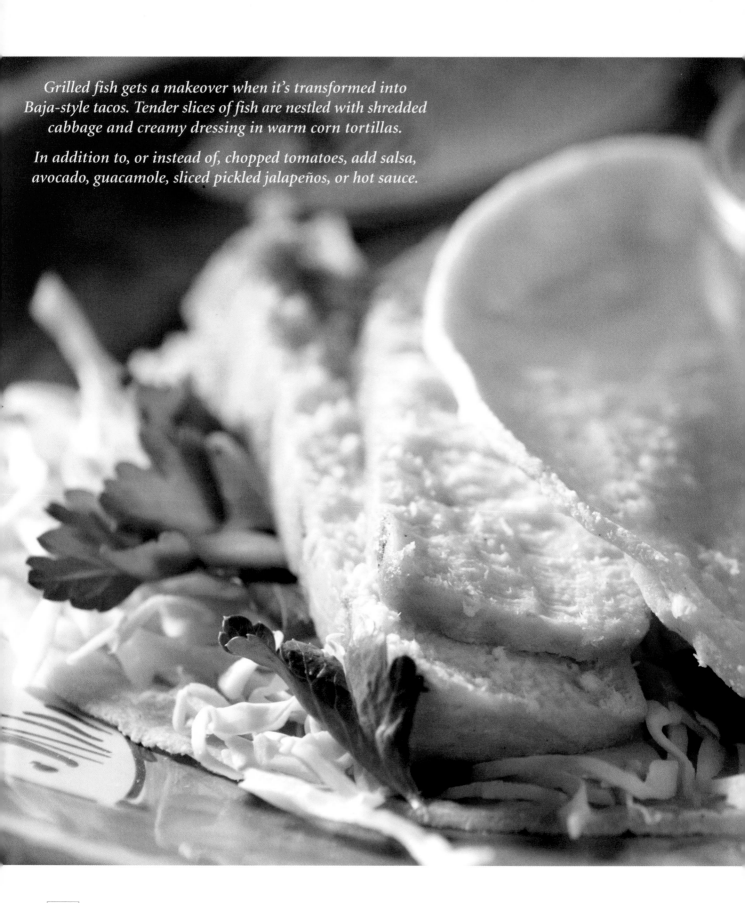

Grilled fish gets a makeover when it's transformed into Baja-style tacos. Tender slices of fish are nestled with shredded cabbage and creamy dressing in warm corn tortillas.

In addition to, or instead of, chopped tomatoes, add salsa, avocado, guacamole, sliced pickled jalapeños, or hot sauce.

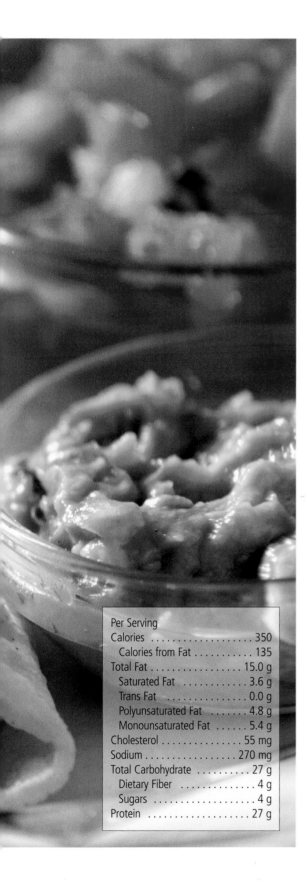

Per Serving	
Calories	350
Calories from Fat	135
Total Fat	15.0 g
Saturated Fat	3.6 g
Trans Fat	0.0 g
Polyunsaturated Fat	4.8 g
Monounsaturated Fat	5.4 g
Cholesterol	55 mg
Sodium	270 mg
Total Carbohydrate	27 g
Dietary Fiber	4 g
Sugars	4 g
Protein	27 g

GRILLED BAJA–STYLE FISH TACOS

SERVES 4 / PREP TIME: 30 MINUTES OR LESS INCLUDING MARINATING
TOTAL TIME: 45 MINUTES OR LESS

1 tablespoon olive oil
2 tablespoons fresh lime juice, divided
1 pound swordfish steak or other hearty white fish fillets
  (such as halibut or cod)
Salt and freshly ground black pepper
1/2 cup chopped fresh cilantro
1/4 cup reduced–fat or regular sour cream
1/4 cup good-quality light mayonnaise, such as Hellmann's
1 jalapeño, seeded and finely chopped
8 (6-inch) corn tortillas
1 cup shredded cabbage or coleslaw mix
1 tomato, chopped, or Fresh Tomato Salsa or Tomatillo Salsa
  (pages 163 and 164)

In a shallow plate, combine oil and 1 tablespoon lime juice. Add fish, turning to coat, and marinate for 15 minutes.

Preheat a lightly oiled grill to medium-high.

Remove fish from marinade and sprinkle with salt and pepper. Grill fish for 4 to 7 minutes per side, or until cooked through. Remove from grill and let rest for 5 minutes before slicing into 1/3- to 1/2-inch thick pieces.

Meanwhile, in a bowl, combine cilantro, sour cream, mayonnaise, jalapeño, and the remaining 1 tablespoon lime juice.

Wrap the tortillas in a damp paper towel and warm in the microwave on HIGH for 15 to 30 seconds.

Top each tortilla with cabbage, sour cream mixture, and fish. Sprinkle with tomatoes.

Serve with Black Bean and Corn Salad (page 115).

MICROWAVE THAI RED CURRY SALMON

Microwaving fish in parchment paper is a quick and easy way to get a delicious meal on the table. Try to find fillets that are of similar thickness for even cooking.

This recipe is easily halved for a single serving.

SERVES 2 / PREP TIME: 15 MINUTES OR LESS / TOTAL TIME: 15 MINUTES OR LESS

½ zucchini, halved lengthwise and very thinly sliced
2 (4-ounce) skinless salmon or thick white fish fillets
1 tablespoon fresh lime juice

1 teaspoon red curry paste
1 garlic clove, minced
2 scallions, white and light green parts only, thinly sliced

Tear off two 10-by-14-inch pieces of parchment paper. Fold in half to make a crease. Place a layer of zucchini to one side of crease on each piece of parchment. Top with salmon.

In a bowl, combine lime juice, curry paste, and garlic. Spread mixture on each fillet and sprinkle with scallions.

Fold over parchment and crimp edges to seal, forming a half-moon shape. Place on a plate. Microwave on HIGH for 3 to 4 minutes, or until the fish flakes. Let stand 2 to 3 minutes. To serve, place parchment packs on individual plates.

Thai red curry paste—a blend of chile peppers, garlic, lemongrass, and galanga root—can be found in the Asian foods section of many supermarkets or specialty markets.

Per Serving
Calories 210
  Calories from Fat 90
Total Fat . . . . 10.0 g
  Saturated Fat . . . . 1.7 g
  Trans Fat . . . . 0.0 g
  Polyunsaturated Fat . . . . 2.2 g
  Monounsaturated Fat . . . . . . 4.7 g
Cholesterol . . . . 75 mg
Sodium . . . . 160 mg
Total Carbohydrate . . . . 4 g
  Dietary Fiber . . . . 1 g
  Sugars . . . . 2 g
Protein . . . . 25 g

GINGER-POACHED SALMON WITH ORANGE AND HONEY

Sweetened with honey and fresh orange juice, with an undertone of gingery spice, this salmon dish is quick enough to whip up on a weeknight, but elegant enough to serve to guests. Pickled ginger, familiar to many as a sushi condiment, is now available at most supermarkets.

SERVES 4 / PREP TIME: 15 MINUTES OR LESS / TOTAL TIME: 30 MINUTES OR LESS

1 orange
1½ cups reduced–sodium chicken broth
2 teaspoons finely chopped fresh
  ginger
2 teaspoons finely chopped pickled
  ginger

2 tablespoons honey
4 salmon fillets (approximately 1 pound),
  preferably skinless
1 tablespoon butter

Grate the zest and squeeze the juice from the orange.

In a large skillet, combine orange zest and juice, chicken broth, both types of ginger, and honey and bring to a boil, stirring to combine. Reduce the heat and simmer for 1 to 2 minutes, stirring frequently. Add salmon, cover, and cook for 4 to 5 minutes per side, or until cooked through. Remove the salmon and keep warm. Increase the heat until the sauce comes to a boil. Whisk in the butter until the sauce thickens to a glaze-like consistency. Pour over the salmon.

Ginger has long been touted as an herbal remedy for stomach distress and other ailments.

Per Serving	
Calories	240
Calories from Fat	90
Total Fat	10.0 g
Saturated Fat	3.2 g
Trans Fat	0.0 g
Polyunsaturated Fat	2.4 g
Monounsaturated Fat	3.2 g
Cholesterol	60 mg
Sodium	265 mg
Total Carbohydrate	12 g
Dietary Fiber	0 g
Sugars	11 g
Protein	25 g

MUSSELS WITH FENNEL, LEEK, AND GRAPE TOMATOES

Mussels are an often-neglected shellfish, but there's no reason they should be! Economical, low in calories, and adaptable to many recipes, there are many reasons to make mussels part of your recipe repertoire. Although mussels used to require lengthy scrubbing and debearding, they are now cultivated for easier preparation.

Use a large stockpot with a tight-fitting lid. Make sure mussel shells are closed before cooking, and discard any that do not open after cooking.

To complete the meal, add a salad and crusty bread for dunking into the yummy vegetable-flecked broth.

SERVES 6 / PREP TIME: 15 MINUTES OR LESS / TOTAL TIME: 30 MINUTES OR LESS

---

2 tablespoons olive oil
4 garlic cloves, minced
1 leek, white and light green part only, sliced
1 fennel bulb, cored and chopped

1½ cups halved grape tomatoes
¼ cup chopped fresh Italian parsley
4 pounds mussels, cleaned and debearded if necessary
1 cup white wine

In a large stockpot over medium heat, add oil. Sauté garlic, leek, and fennel for 8 to 10 minutes, or until softened. Add tomatoes and parsley and stir to combine. Add wine and increase heat to high. Add the mussels, cover, and cook for 5 to 8 minutes, or until mussels have opened, shaking the pot once or twice during cooking.

If any mussels do not open, return them to the pan. If they still don't open after 1 to 2 minutes, discard.

Mussels have nearly three times as much iron as most meats and are a good source of zinc.
. . . . .
Before cooking, wash mussels to remove any debris and pull off any fibrous "beards." Discard any mussels with broken shells or if shells are open and don't close when you tap them.

Per Serving	
Calories	235
Calories from Fat	80
Total Fat	9.0 g
Saturated Fat	1.4 g
Trans Fat	0.0 g
Polyunsaturated Fat	1.6 g
Monounsaturated Fat	4.2 g
Cholesterol	50 mg
Sodium	350 mg
Total Carbohydrate	14 g
Dietary Fiber	2 g
Sugars	9 g
Protein	22 g

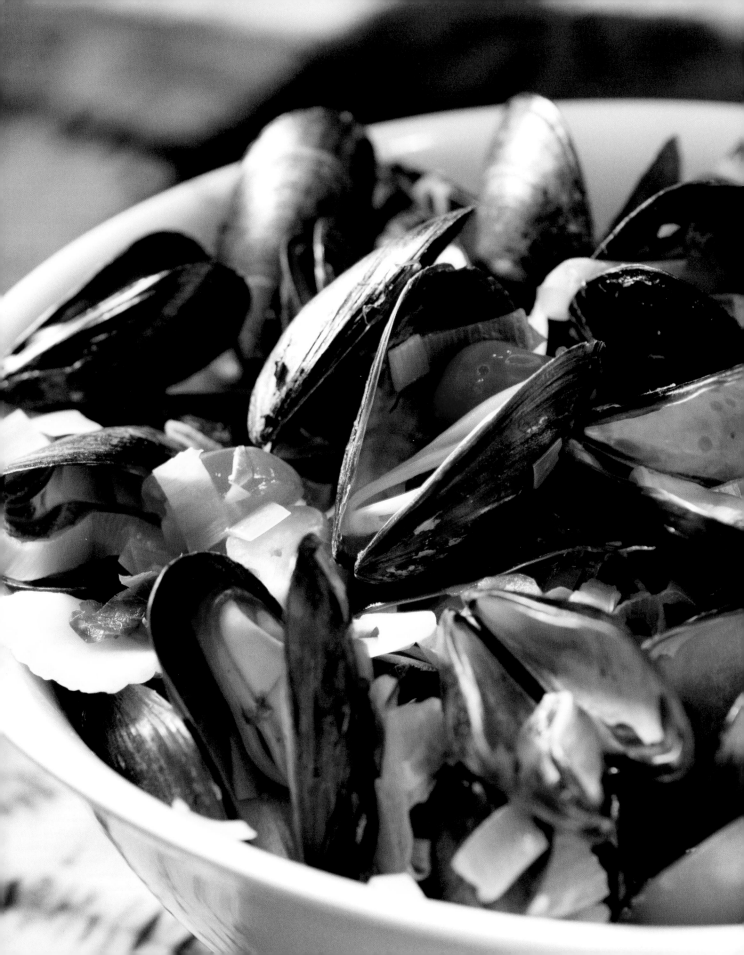

TOMATO–FENNEL TOFU BAKE

Don't be intimidated by the long list of ingredients—everything is just thrown into a casserole dish for this savory, satisfying one-pot supper. Even the rice is added without precooking.

If not using basmati, your rice might cook faster, so check for doneness at the 15-minute intervals.

SERVES 4 / PREP TIME: 15 MINUTES OR LESS / TOTAL TIME: 2 HOURS OR LESS

1 tablespoon olive oil

1 cup brown basmati rice

4 garlic cloves, minced

1 (14- to 16-ounce) block extra-firm tofu, drained and patted dry

8 ounces sliced cremini ("baby bella") mushrooms

1 fennel bulb, quartered, cored, and sliced crosswise

2 leeks, white and light green parts only, halved lengthwise and thinly sliced crosswise

2 cups fresh spinach, thinly sliced

1/2 cup sun-dried tomatoes (not oil-packed), julienned

1/2 teaspoon fennel seeds

1/4 teaspoon anise seeds

1/4 teaspoon crushed red pepper flakes

1 teaspoon dried basil

1/2 teaspoon freshly ground black pepper

1 teaspoon salt

1/4 cup plus 2 tablespoons tomato paste

3 to 4 cups reduced–sodium chicken broth or vegetable broth

Preheat the oven to 350 degrees.

In a 3-quart casserole dish with a cover, combine oil and uncooked rice, stirring to coat rice and the bottom of the dish. Stir in garlic. Cut the tofu into quarters, then into 1/2-inch thick slices. Place over rice and top with mushrooms, fennel, leeks, spinach, and sun-dried tomatoes. Sprinkle with fennel seeds, anise seeds, red pepper flakes, basil, black pepper, and salt. Stir together the tomato paste and 3 cups broth and pour over all the vegetables.

Cover the casserole and bake for 30 minutes. Remove from the oven and gently stir the contents to combine and moisten them. Cover and return to the oven and bake for 50 to 60 minutes, stirring gently every 15 minutes, adding more broth if necessary, until the rice is tender and most of the liquid has been absorbed. Cool for 10 to 15 minutes before serving. Season with salt and pepper.

Per Serving	
Calories	380
Calories from Fat	65
Total Fat	7.0 g
Saturated Fat	1.2 g
Trans Fat	0.0 g
Polyunsaturated Fat	2.2 g
Monounsaturated Fat	3.5 g
Cholesterol	0 mg
Sodium	1090 mg
Total Carbohydrate	62 g
Dietary Fiber	9 g
Sugars	9 g
Protein	18 g

TANDOORI-STYLE CHICKEN

A great way to infuse flavor without adding a lot of fat is to marinate chicken in a spiced yogurt mixture before baking it. The marinade bathes the chicken, keeping it moist, while Indian spices, including cumin, coriander, and turmeric, penetrate deep into the meat.

Put the chicken in to marinate before leaving for work, and when you get home all you need to do is bake it. The chicken can also be grilled.

To lower the calories and fat, remove the skin from the chicken after cooking, or buy skinless chicken pieces (with the bone still in) instead of using a whole cut-up chicken.

SERVES 6 / PREP TIME: 15 MINUTES OR LESS
TOTAL TIME: 1 HOUR OR LESS PLUS 4 TO 24 HOURS TO MARINATE

---

2 garlic cloves
$\frac{1}{4}$ cup fresh cilantro
1 small jalapeño, stemmed and seeded
1-inch piece fresh ginger, peeled
$\frac{1}{2}$ onion, quartered
1 cup nonfat plain yogurt
2 teaspoons ground cumin

2 teaspoons ground coriander
1 teaspoon salt
$\frac{1}{2}$ teaspoon ground turmeric, optional
$\frac{1}{4}$ teaspoon cayenne pepper
1 (3$\frac{1}{2}$- to 4-pound) chicken, cut into 8 pieces
1 teaspoon canola oil

In a food processor with the motor running, add garlic. Add cilantro, jalapeño, ginger, and onion and pulse until coarsely chopped. Add yogurt, cumin, coriander, salt, turmeric, and cayenne pepper and pulse to combine, scraping down sides to blend. Transfer to a bowl or zip-top bag.

With a sharp knife, slash chicken diagonally along the grain, about $\frac{1}{2}$ inch deep and 1 inch apart. Add chicken to marinade and turn pieces to coat. Refrigerate for 4 to 24 hours.

When ready to cook, preheat the oven to 450 degrees.

Remove chicken pieces from marinade and place in a roasting pan. Drizzle with oil.

Bake for 30 to 40 minutes, or until cooked through.

This makes a great meal for entertaining; the chicken can be served hot from the oven or at room temperature. Serve with Basmati Rice and Chickpea Pilaf (page 119).

Per Serving	
Calories	265
Calories from Fat	135
Total Fat	15.0 g
Saturated Fat	4.0 g
Trans Fat	0.0 g
Polyunsaturated Fat	3.3 g
Monounsaturated Fat	6.0 g
Cholesterol	90 mg
Sodium	190 mg
Total Carbohydrate	2 g
Dietary Fiber	0 g
Sugars	1 g
Protein	29 g

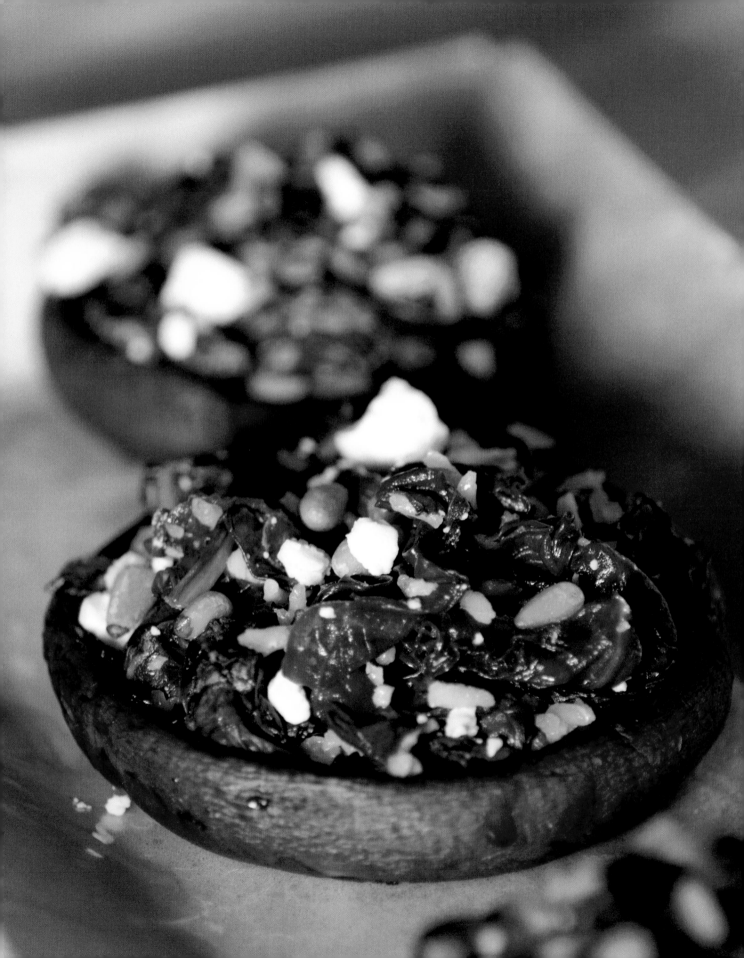

PORTOBELLOS STUFFED WITH SPINACH, BROWN RICE, AND FETA

Meaty portobellos are the perfect vessels for a filling of sautéed spinach, brown rice, and feta cheese. This substantial vegetarian meal combines a variety of flavors and textures to make a satisfying entrée. Just add a salad to round out the meal. To make things even easier, many supermarkets now sell cooked brown rice in pouches, saving a lot of time.

Line your baking sheet with aluminum foil or parchment paper to speed cleanup.

SERVES 4 / PREP TIME: 15 MINUTES OR LESS / TOTAL TIME: 30 MINUTES OR LESS

---

4 large portobello mushroom caps, gills and stems removed
2 tablespoons olive oil
2 garlic cloves, minced
1 shallot, finely chopped
1 (9- or 10-ounce) bag baby spinach

1 cup cooked brown rice
½ cup crumbled feta cheese
1 tablespoon pine nuts, toasted
1 tablespoon fresh lemon juice
Salt and freshly ground black pepper

Preheat the oven to 400 degrees. Lightly coat a baking sheet with nonstick cooking spray.

Lightly brush mushrooms with oil and place rounded side down on the baking sheet.

In a large skillet over medium-high heat, add the remaining oil. Sauté the garlic and shallot for 1 to 2 minutes, or until softened. Add spinach and sauté until bright green and wilted. Add rice and stir to combine. Remove from heat and stir in feta and pine nuts. Season with lemon juice, salt, and pepper and stuff into mushroom caps.

Bake for 10 to 12 minutes, or until cheese melts and mushrooms are heated through.

Toasting nuts brings out their flavor. To toast pine nuts, cook in a dry skillet, shaking frequently, until golden and aromatic, or bake at 350 degrees for 3 to 8 minutes, stirring occasionally. Cool before using.

Per Serving	
Calories	215
Calories from Fat	115
Total Fat	13.0 g
Saturated Fat	3.9 g
Trans Fat	0.2 g
Polyunsaturated Fat	1.9 g
Monounsaturated Fat	6.4 g
Cholesterol	15 mg
Sodium	265 mg
Total Carbohydrate	19 g
Dietary Fiber	3 g
Sugars	2 g
Protein	8 g

OLÉ PASTA CASSEROLE

Ground turkey breast or beef, spicy tomatoes, and a hearty corn and black bean mixture are this dish's signature ingredients. Think "nachos meets pasta" in perfect harmony. Choose the canned tomato variety that matches your spice preference.

SERVES 6 / PREP TIME: 15 MINUTES OR LESS / TOTAL TIME: 45 MINUTES OR LESS

8 ounces whole wheat or regular rotini or other shaped pasta

¾ pound ground turkey breast or lean ground beef

2 (10-ounce) cans diced tomatoes with chiles, such as Ro*Tel

1 (15-ounce) can black beans, rinsed and drained

1 (15-ounce) can no-salt-added corn, drained

½ cup "Mexican-style" shredded cheese

⅓ cup crushed tortilla chips

Preheat the oven to 350 degrees. Lightly coat an 8-by-8-inch baking pan with nonstick cooking spray.

Prepare pasta according to package directions for al dente (just firm). Drain and set aside.

Meanwhile, in a large skillet over medium-high heat, brown the meat for 6 to 8 minutes, stirring frequently to break it up. Drain if necessary. Add tomatoes and their juice, beans, corn, and pasta and stir well to combine. Transfer to baking pan and top with cheese and tortilla crumbs.

Bake for 15 to 20 minutes.

Per Serving	
Calories	350
Calories from Fat	55
Total Fat	6.0 g
Saturated Fat	2.2 g
Trans Fat	0.0 g
Polyunsaturated Fat	0.9 g
Monounsaturated Fat	1.8 g
Cholesterol	45 mg
Sodium	565 mg
Total Carbohydrate	51 g
Dietary Fiber	10 g
Sugars	8 g
Protein	26 g

TASTY TURKEY TACOS

Ground turkey breast and lots of healthy topping options, including shredded lettuce and chopped tomatoes, make this not-too-spicy take on tacos a healthy family treat.

SERVES 6 / PREP TIME: 15 MINUTES OR LESS / TOTAL TIME: 45 MINUTES OR LESS

1 tablespoon canola oil
1 small onion, finely chopped
2 garlic cloves, minced
1¼ pounds ground turkey breast
1 (8-ounce) can tomato sauce
2½ teaspoons chili powder
1½ teaspoons ground cumin
½ teaspoon paprika
Hot sauce, such as Tabasco
Salt and freshly ground black pepper
12 (6-inch) flour tortillas

Optional Toppings:
2 cups shredded lettuce
1 cup chopped tomato
¾ cup "Mexican-style" shredded cheese
½ cup reduced–fat or regular sour cream
½ cup finely chopped red onion
¼ cup chopped jalapeños
Taco sauce or salsa

In a large skillet over medium-high heat, add oil. Sauté the onion for 5 to 8 minutes, or until softened. Add garlic and sauté for 1 minute. Add turkey and cook for 6 to 8 minutes, stirring frequently to break it up. Add tomato sauce, chili powder, cumin, and paprika and stir well to combine. Reduce the heat to low and cook for 8 to 10 minutes, stirring occasionally. Season with hot sauce, salt, and pepper.

Meanwhile, wrap the tortillas in a damp paper towel and warm in the microwave on HIGH for 15 to 30 seconds.

When ready to serve, place toppings in small bowls on the table. Layer about ⅓ cup of turkey in a tortilla and add desired toppings.

Tortillas can also be warmed in an oven set to 250 degrees. Wrap in foil and warm while preparing the filling.
. . . . .
If you want to add more fiber to your diet, choose corn instead of flour tortillas.

Per Serving
Calories 370
   Calories from Fat 80
Total Fat . . . . 9.0 g
   Saturated Fat . . . . 1.7 g
   Trans Fat . . . . 0.0 g
   Polyunsaturated Fat . . . . 2.1 g
   Monounsaturated Fat . . . . . . 4.4 g
Cholesterol . . . . 60 mg
Sodium . . . . 735 mg
Total Carbohydrate . . . . 43 g
   Dietary Fiber . . . . 3 g
   Sugars . . . . 4 g
Protein . . . . 29 g

GREEN CURRY SHRIMP

A restaurant Thai green curry is usually a caloric bonanza, drowning in high-fat coconut milk and oil. Making your own version allows you to load it with veggies and healthful protein and make smart substitutions, like "lite" coconut milk. Unsweetened "lite" coconut milk, located in the international section of most supermarkets, has 65% less fat than its regular counterpart.

Curry paste, also available in most supermarkets or by mail order, provides authentic flavor. Thai curry pastes have a lot of concentrated flavor. Start with the minimum amount and add more, depending on your spice preference.

Serve over rice or soba noodles.

SERVES 4 / PREP TIME: 15 MINUTES OR LESS / TOTAL TIME: 30 MINUTES OR LESS

¾ cup "lite" coconut milk, well shaken

½ to 1 teaspoon green curry paste, or to taste

1 tablespoon canola oil

1 red bell pepper, seeded and thinly sliced

1 cup stemmed, sliced shiitake mushrooms

1 pound peeled and deveined shrimp

1 cup green beans, cut into 1-inch pieces

½ cup frozen peas

1 tablespoon fish sauce

2 tablespoons sliced fresh basil, optional

In a bowl, combine coconut milk and ½ teaspoon curry paste.

In a wok or large skillet over high heat, add oil. Sauté the bell pepper and mushrooms for 2 to 5 minutes, or until softened. Add shrimp and green beans and sauté for 1 to 2 minutes. Add curry mixture, peas, fish sauce, and basil. Cover and simmer for 3 to 4 minutes, or until shrimp are cooked through. Taste and adjust seasoning as desired.

Per Serving	
Calories	185
Calories from Fat	65
Total Fat	7.0 g
Saturated Fat	2.0 g
Trans Fat	0.0 g
Polyunsaturated Fat	1.6 g
Monounsaturated Fat	2.6 g
Cholesterol	160 mg
Sodium	680 mg
Total Carbohydrate	10 g
Dietary Fiber	3 g
Sugars	4 g
Protein	20 g

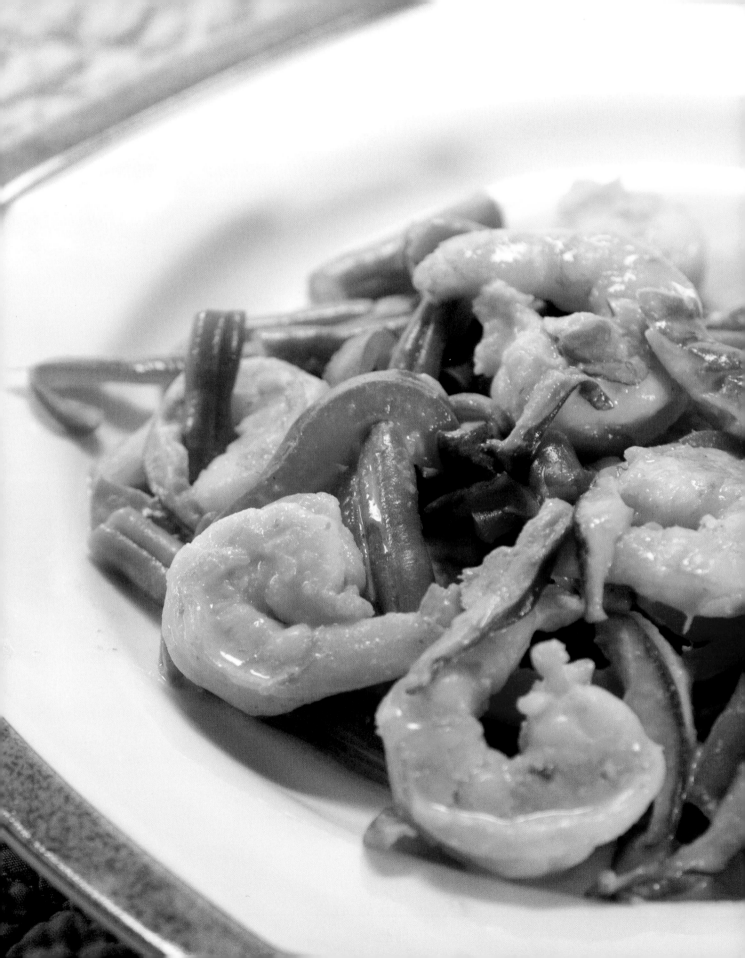

LOWER-FAT MAC-N-CHEESE

Low-fat milk and reduced-fat cheddar cheese lessen the calories but not the taste in this version of the creamy classic. You can serve it right out of the saucepan or baked in a casserole topped with bread crumbs and Parmesan cheese.

For a grown-up twist, layer tomato slices under the crumb topping.

SERVES 4 / PREP TIME: 15 MINUTES OR LESS / TOTAL TIME: 45 MINUTES OR LESS

8 ounces elbow macaroni
1 tablespoon butter
1 tablespoon all-purpose flour
1 cup low-fat (1%) milk
8 ounces reduced-fat cheddar cheese,
  such as Cabot of VT 50% light,
  shredded

1 tomato, sliced, optional
3 tablespoons plain bread crumbs
1 tablespoon freshly grated Parmesan
  cheese

Preheat the oven to 400 degrees. Lightly coat an 8-by-8-inch baking pan with nonstick cooking spray.

Prepare macaroni according to package directions for al dente (just firm). Drain and set aside.

Meanwhile, in a saucepan over medium heat, melt the butter. Whisk in the flour until completely incorporated, 20 to 30 seconds. Add milk and cook until thickened and starting to bubble around the edges, whisking to incorporate the flour mixture. Reduce the heat, add the cheddar cheese, and cook, stirring constantly, until melted and thickened. Add pasta and stir well to combine.

Transfer to baking pan, top with tomatoes, and sprinkle with bread crumbs and Parmesan cheese. Lightly coat the top with nonstick cooking spray.

Bake for 10 to 15 minutes.

> If you're using reduced-fat cheese, choose "sharp" varieties for extra flavor.

Per Serving	
Calories	435
Calories from Fat	125
Total Fat	14.0 g
Saturated Fat	8.5 g
Trans Fat	0.0 g
Polyunsaturated Fat	1.1 g
Monounsaturated Fat	3.9 g
Cholesterol	45 mg
Sodium	445 mg
Total Carbohydrate	51 g
Dietary Fiber	2 g
Sugars	6 g
Protein	27 g

APRICOT–ORANGE BAKED CHICKEN

*This company-worthy dish uses a cut-up whole chicken
for an elegant but economical meal.*

Serve with brown rice or another grain to absorb the delicious pan juices.

SERVES 6 / PREP TIME: 15 MINUTES OR LESS / TOTAL TIME: 1 HOUR OR LESS

1 (3½- to 4-pound) chicken, cut into
  8 pieces
Salt and freshly ground black pepper
⅓ cup apricot preserves
½ cup orange juice

½ cup reduced–sodium chicken broth
½ cup dried apricots
2 tablespoons currants or raisins
2 tablespoons light brown sugar

Preheat the oven to 375 degrees.

In a 13-by-9-inch baking pan, place chicken in a single layer. Sprinkle with salt and pepper.

In a bowl, combine apricot preserves and orange juice. Brush chicken pieces with mixture. Add chicken broth to the remaining mixture and pour into pan.

Bake for 20 minutes. Remove from the oven and add apricots and currants. Sprinkle the chicken evenly with brown sugar. Bake for 30 to 40 minutes, or until chicken is shiny, golden, and cooked through.

To lower the calories and fat, remove the skin from the chicken after cooking, or buy skinless chicken pieces (with the bones still in) instead of using a whole cut-up chicken. Removing the skin in this recipe saves 85 calories and 8 grams of fat per serving!

Per Serving
Calories 355
  Calories from Fat 125
Total Fat . . . . 14.0 g
  Saturated Fat . . . . 3.9 g
  Trans Fat . . . . 0.0 g
  Polyunsaturated Fat . . . . 3.1 g
  Monounsaturated Fat . . . . . . 5.6 g
Cholesterol . . . . 90 mg
Sodium . . . . 140 mg
Total Carbohydrate . . . . 28 g
  Dietary Fiber . . . . 1 g
  Sugars . . . . 24 g
Protein . . . . 29 g

CRUNCHY "OVEN-FRIED" CHICKEN NUGGETS

Kids and adults will love this healthful rendition of chicken nuggets.
The coating adds a big crunch and keeps the meat tender and moist.
Who knew nuggets could be so good...and good for you!

Line your baking sheet with aluminum foil or parchment paper to speed cleanup.

SERVES 4 / PREP TIME: 15 MINUTES OR LESS / TOTAL TIME: 30 MINUTES OR LESS

---

10 classic or whole grain Melba toasts
 (2 pouches)
1 tablespoon canola oil
1 egg
1 teaspoon Dijon mustard

1/4 teaspoon dried oregano
1/4 teaspoon salt
1/4 teaspoon garlic powder
1 pound boneless, skinless chicken
 breasts, cut into 2-inch "nuggets"

Preheat the oven to 400 degrees. Place a cooling rack on a rimmed baking sheet.

In a food processor, pulse the Melba toast until pieces are about 1/8 inch in size, with some smaller and larger pieces. Don't overprocess. Add oil and pulse once or twice, or until crumbs are just moistened. (You can also use a rolling pin or a meat mallet to crush the toasts in a zip-top bag. Then mix the oil and crumbs together in a bowl.) Transfer crumbs to a plate.

In a bowl, beat egg. Add mustard, oregano, salt, and garlic powder and beat to combine. Dip chicken in egg mixture, then in crumbs, pressing to coat all sides of the meat. Place on the rack.

Bake for 15 minutes, or until cooked through.

Canola oil (and olive oil, too) is high in oleic acid, a monounsaturated fatty acid that can help reduce low-density lipoproteins (or LDL—the "bad cholesterol") without lowering high-density lipoproteins (or HDL—the "good cholesterol").

Per Serving	
Calories	230
Calories from Fat	70
Total Fat	8.0 g
Saturated Fat	1.5 g
Trans Fat	0.0 g
Polyunsaturated Fat	2.0 g
Monounsaturated Fat	3.6 g
Cholesterol	120 mg
Sodium	355 mg
Total Carbohydrate	10 g
Dietary Fiber	1 g
Sugars	0 g
Protein	27 g

STEAMED PESTO-ROLLED TILAPIA WITH VEGETABLES

This guest-worthy entrée is actually a snap to prepare, thanks to refrigerated store-bought pesto. The veggies add a burst of color and flavor, in addition to a variety of nutrients. If desired, drizzle with olive oil before serving.

SERVES 4 / PREP TIME: 15 MINUTES OR LESS / TOTAL TIME: 30 MINUTES OR LESS

4 tilapia fillets
Salt and freshly ground black pepper
2 tablespoons pesto
1 red bell pepper, seeded and thinly sliced

1 cup stemmed, thinly sliced shiitake mushrooms
1 cup matchstick-cut carrots

Lightly season tilapia with salt and pepper. Spread a very thin layer of pesto on top of each fillet. Roll up the fillets and tie with kitchen twine or skewer with toothpicks to hold each roll in place.

Lightly coat a steamer basket with nonstick cooking spray. Set the basket in a large stockpot with water filled to just below the basket. Add fish rolls and surround with bell pepper, mushrooms, and carrots. Place over medium-high heat, cover, and cook for 8 to 10 minutes, or until fish is cooked through and vegetables are tender. Serve fish with vegetables.

This dish is a delicious way to add more vegetables to your day. Don't limit yourself just to the vegetables mentioned. Add julienned zucchini or beets, green beans, or broccoli florets.

Per Serving
Calories 165
  Calories from Fat 45
Total Fat . . . . 5.0 g
  Saturated Fat . . . . 1.5 g
  Trans Fat . . . . 0.0 g
  Polyunsaturated Fat . . . . 1.0 g
  Monounsaturated Fat . . . . . . 2.2 g
Cholesterol . . . . 75 mg
Sodium . . . . 90 mg
Total Carbohydrate . . . . 7 g
  Dietary Fiber . . . . 2 g
  Sugars . . . . 3 g
Protein . . . . 24 g

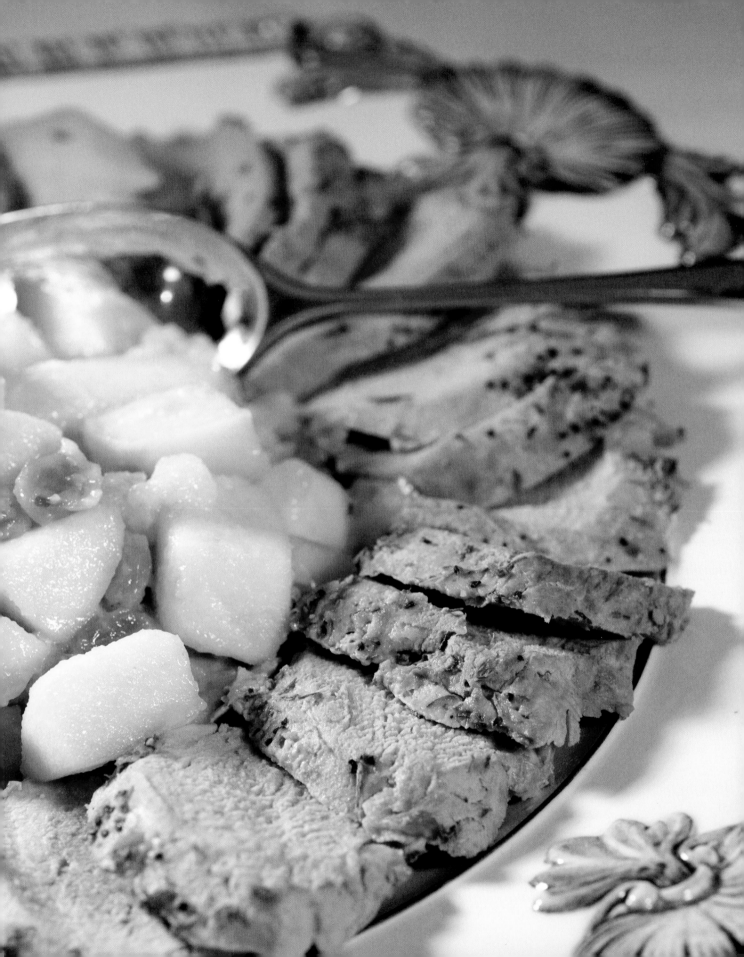

PORK TENDERLOIN TOPPED WITH FALL FRUITS

Roasted pork tenderloin is topped with a chunky blend of fruits, including pears and apples. The sweetness of the fruit is the perfect counterpoint to the pork.

Line your baking sheet with aluminum foil or parchment paper to speed cleanup.

SERVES 6 / PREP TIME: 15 MINUTES OR LESS / TOTAL TIME: 45 MINUTES OR LESS

1 tablespoon Dijon mustard

2 teaspoons dried thyme

2 pork tenderloins (about 1½ pounds), trimmed of excess fat and silverskin

Salt and freshly ground black pepper

2 teaspoons canola oil

2 ripe firm pears, peeled, cored, and cut into 1-inch pieces

2 Golden Delicious apples, peeled, cored, and cut into 1-inch pieces

1 tablespoon finely chopped fresh ginger

¼ cup golden raisins

¼ to ½ cup apple cider or juice

Preheat the oven to 450 degrees. Lightly coat a rimmed baking sheet with nonstick cooking spray.

In a bowl, combine mustard and thyme. Sprinkle the pork with salt and pepper and cover with mustard mixture. Place pork on the baking sheet.

Bake for 20 to 25 minutes, or until an instant-read thermometer registers 155 degrees. Let rest for 5 minutes before slicing.

Meanwhile, in a skillet over medium-high heat, add oil. Sauté the pears, apples, and ginger for 5 minutes, or until lightly colored. Add raisins and ¼ cup apple cider. Reduce the heat, cover, and simmer for 10 minutes, or until fruit is tender, stirring occasionally. If more liquid is needed, add the remaining juice, 1 tablespoon at a time.

Slice tenderloins and top with fruit mixture.

Per Serving	
Calories	210
Calories from Fat	45
Total Fat	5.0 g
Saturated Fat	1.1 g
Trans Fat	0.0 g
Polyunsaturated Fat	0.8 g
Monounsaturated Fat	2.1 g
Cholesterol	60 mg
Sodium	105 mg
Total Carbohydrate	21 g
Dietary Fiber	3 g
Sugars	16 g
Protein	22 g

CHICKEN CHILI

Get the satisfaction of a hearty bowl of chili with a lot less fat and effort.
This "white" chili is filled with veggies, beans, and chunks of chicken breast.

SERVES 4 / PREP TIME: 30 MINUTES OR LESS / TOTAL TIME: 1 HOUR OR LESS

---

1 tablespoon canola oil
1 onion, chopped
1 red bell pepper, seeded and chopped
1 jalapeño, seeded and finely chopped
2 garlic cloves, minced
2 tablespoons chili powder
2 teaspoons ground cumin
1 teaspoon dried oregano
$\frac{1}{2}$ teaspoon salt

$\frac{1}{4}$ teaspoon cayenne pepper, optional
1 pound boneless, skinless chicken
breasts or thighs, cut into $\frac{1}{2}$-inch pieces
1 (14$\frac{1}{2}$-ounce) can reduced–sodium
chicken broth
1 (14$\frac{1}{2}$-ounce) can diced tomatoes
2 (15-ounce) cans cannellini or navy
beans, rinsed and drained

In a stockpot over medium heat, add oil. Sauté the onion, bell pepper, jalapeño, and garlic for 8 to 10 minutes, or until softened. Add chili powder, cumin, oregano, salt, and cayenne pepper and stir to combine. Add chicken and cook for 3 to 5 minutes, stirring frequently.

Add broth and tomatoes and their juice and bring to a boil, stirring to combine. Reduce the heat, cover, and simmer for 10 to 15 minutes, stirring occasionally. Add beans and simmer, uncovered, for 15 to 20 minutes, or until thickened, stirring occasionally.

Canola oil is trans fat- and cholesterol-free and is the lowest in saturated fat of any common edible oil.

. . . . .

Beans are an easy and healthy choice to add more fiber to your day. Good-quality canned beans are as good as using cooked dried beans, and much faster.

Per Serving	
Calories	420
Calories from Fat	70
Total Fat	8.0 g
Saturated Fat	1.2 g
Trans Fat	0.0 g
Polyunsaturated Fat	2.6 g
Monounsaturated Fat	3.4 g
Cholesterol	65 mg
Sodium	990 mg
Total Carbohydrate	48 g
Dietary Fiber	13 g
Sugars	8 g
Protein	40 g

CHICKEN AND BARLEY STEW

This healthful and flavorful stew combines an assortment of vegetables with barley, a nutritious grain that provides protein, B vitamins, potassium, and fiber with very little sodium or fat. Studies have shown that this wonder grain also fights cholesterol production. A touch of fresh dill makes the stew sing.

SERVES 6 / PREP TIME: 30 MINUTES OR LESS / TOTAL TIME: 1 HOUR AND 15 MINUTES OR LESS

1 tablespoon canola oil
2 carrots, chopped
2 celery stalks, chopped
2 garlic cloves, minced
1 onion, chopped
1 cup sliced mushrooms
1 cup stemmed, sliced shiitake
   mushrooms

5 cups reduced–sodium chicken broth
1 (14½-ounce) can diced tomatoes
   (preferably petite cut), drained
1 cup pearl barley
1 pound boneless, skinless chicken
   breasts, cut into ½-inch pieces
1 tablespoon fresh dill
Salt and freshly ground black pepper

In a large stockpot over medium-high heat, add oil. Sauté the carrots, celery, garlic, onion, and both types of mushrooms until softened, 8 to 10 minutes, stirring frequently.

Add broth and tomatoes and bring to a boil, stirring to combine. Add barley and stir to combine. Reduce the heat, cover, and simmer for 30 to 40 minutes, stirring occasionally, or until the barley is tender and the stew thickens. Add chicken and dill and cook for 5 to 7 minutes, or until the chicken is cooked through. Season with salt and pepper.

Have chicken stock left over after making a recipe? An easy way to store leftover chicken broth is to pour it into ice cube trays and freeze. Once frozen, keep in a freezer bag and take out cubes as needed.

Per Serving	
Calories	290
Calories from Fat	45
Total Fat	5.0 g
Saturated Fat	0.8 g
Trans Fat	0.0 g
Polyunsaturated Fat	1.4 g
Monounsaturated Fat	2.1 g
Cholesterol	45 mg
Sodium	570 mg
Total Carbohydrate	41 g
Dietary Fiber	6 g
Sugars	5 g
Protein	22 g

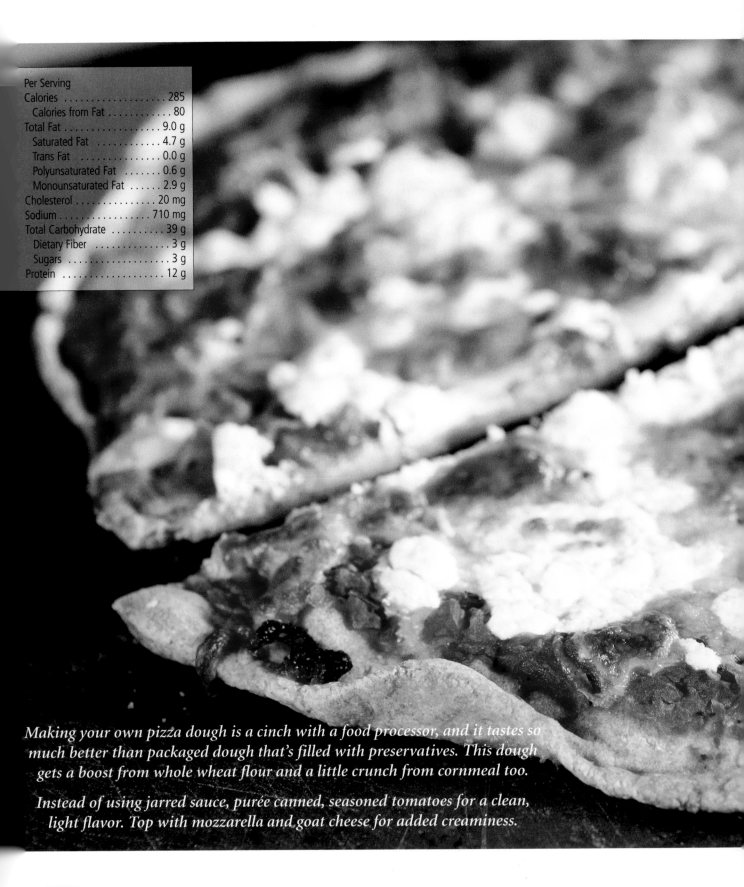

Per Serving
Calories 285
  Calories from Fat 80
Total Fat . . . . 9.0 g
  Saturated Fat . . . . 4.7 g
  Trans Fat . . . . 0.0 g
  Polyunsaturated Fat . . . . 0.6 g
  Monounsaturated Fat . . . . . . 2.9 g
Cholesterol . . . . 20 mg
Sodium . . . . 710 mg
Total Carbohydrate . . . . 39 g
  Dietary Fiber . . . . 3 g
  Sugars . . . . 3 g
Protein . . . . 12 g

Making your own pizza dough is a cinch with a food processor, and it tastes so much better than packaged dough that's filled with preservatives. This dough gets a boost from whole wheat flour and a little crunch from cornmeal too.

Instead of using jarred sauce, purée canned, seasoned tomatoes for a clean, light flavor. Top with mozzarella and goat cheese for added creaminess.

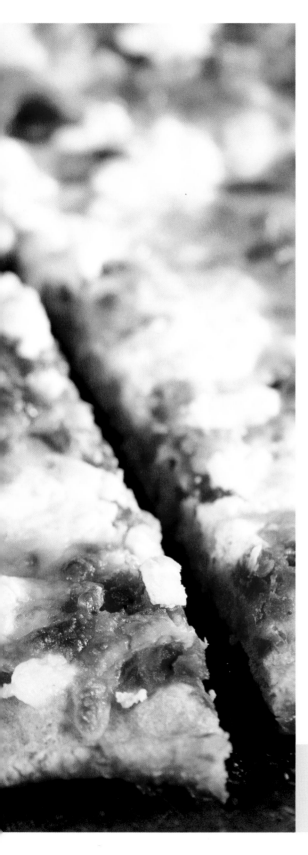

HOMEMADE PIZZA

MAKES 2 (11-INCH) PIZZAS (8 SERVINGS) / PREP TIME: 30 MINUTES OR LESS
TOTAL TIME: 2 HOURS OR LESS INCLUDING RISING TIME

1 package (2$\frac{1}{2}$ teaspoons) active dry yeast
1 cup warm water (about 110 degrees)
Pinch granulated sugar
2 cups flour (all-purpose, bread, or combination)
$\frac{3}{4}$ cup whole wheat flour
$\frac{1}{4}$ cup cornmeal
1 teaspoon salt
1 tablespoon olive oil, plus extra for greasing the bowl
2 (14$\frac{1}{2}$-ounce) cans diced tomatoes with basil, garlic, and oregano
1 cup shredded part-skim mozzarella cheese
4 ounces goat cheese, crumbled

In a food processor, sprinkle the yeast over warm water. Add sugar and let stand 5 minutes to dissolve. Add both flours, cornmeal, salt, and oil and process until the dough forms a ball, becoming smooth and cleaning the sides of the bowl.

Transfer dough to a lightly oiled bowl and rotate to coat all sides. Cover the bowl with plastic wrap or a clean cloth and leave it to double in size, about 1 hour.

When the dough has risen, preheat the oven to 450 degrees. Turn dough out onto a lightly floured surface. Punch down and knead briefly to deflate. Let it rest for 15 minutes. Divide in half. On a lightly floured surface, roll or stretch the dough to desired size. Coat a baking sheet or pizza pan lightly with cornmeal to prevent sticking, and place the dough on the pan.

Meanwhile, in a food processor, pulse tomatoes until small dice. Drain of excess liquid and divide on crusts. Sprinkle with mozzarella and goat cheese.

Bake for 12 to 18 minutes, or until cheeses melt.

Few would think of pizza as health food, but if you go heavy on tomatoes and veggie toppings, rather than meat and cheese, you'll save calories and fat and get the benefits of lycopene and other disease-fighting antioxidants!

WHOLE WHEAT PENNE WITH ROASTED VEGETABLE SAUCE

Roasting brings out vegetables' natural sugars and gives them a delicious caramelized flavor. Just pop the baking sheet in the oven and let the heat do the rest. With very little effort, vegetables can be used to create a luscious sauce that can stand up to whole wheat pasta.

Line your baking sheet with aluminum foil or parchment paper to speed cleanup.

SERVES 8 / PREP TIME: 15 MINUTES OR LESS / TOTAL TIME: 1 HOUR OR LESS

---

3 tablespoons olive oil
4 plum tomatoes, cut into 1-inch pieces
4 garlic cloves, halved
2 red bell peppers, seeded and cut into 1-inch pieces
1 eggplant, peeled and cut into 1-inch pieces

1 red onion, cut into 1-inch pieces
Salt and freshly ground black pepper
1 cup reduced–sodium chicken broth or vegetable broth, heated
1 pound whole wheat penne
1 tablespoon thinly sliced fresh basil, optional

Preheat the oven to 400 degrees. Brush a rimmed baking sheet lightly with oil.

Combine tomatoes, garlic, bell peppers, eggplant, and onion on the baking sheet. Drizzle with the remaining oil and sprinkle generously with salt and pepper. Toss to combine and spread out evenly over sheet.

Roast for 45 minutes, or until vegetables are tender and slightly charred, stirring every 15 to 20 minutes.

Transfer vegetables to a food processor and add broth. Blend until smooth, adding additional broth to achieve desired consistency.

Meanwhile, prepare penne according to package directions for al dente (just firm) and drain.

In a serving bowl, combine pasta and sauce and garnish with basil.

> Whole grains have more nutrients—including fiber—than refined grains. A 2-ounce serving of whole wheat pasta provides 5 to 7 grams of fiber, compared with only 2 grams for pasta made with refined flour.

Per Serving	
Calories	295
Calories from Fat	55
Total Fat	6.0 g
Saturated Fat	0.9 g
Trans Fat	0.0 g
Polyunsaturated Fat	1.0 g
Monounsaturated Fat	3.9 g
Cholesterol	0 mg
Sodium	70 mg
Total Carbohydrate	55 g
Dietary Fiber	9 g
Sugars	7 g
Protein	9 g

CHICKEN AND BROCCOLI STIR-FRY

The beauty of a stir-fry is its adaptability. Feel free to substitute your favorite vegetables, protein, and sauce. Just remember to load this dish with a variety of veggies and add them in order of cooking time needed. Allow an extra minute or two for larger pieces or denser vegetables.

Serve over brown rice or soba noodles.

SERVES 4 / PREP TIME: 15 MINUTES OR LESS / TOTAL TIME: 30 MINUTES OR LESS

1 tablespoon canola oil
5 cups or 1 (12-ounce) bag broccoli
   florets
3 garlic cloves, thinly sliced
¼ cup water
¾ pound boneless, skinless chicken
   breasts, cut into thin strips

1 yellow bell pepper, seeded and cut
   into 1-inch pieces
1 (8-ounce) can water chestnuts,
   drained
⅓ cup stir-fry sauce

In a wok or large skillet over high heat, add oil. Sauté the broccoli and garlic for 1 minute. Add water and cook for 3 to 5 minutes, or until broccoli turns bright green, stirring frequently. Add chicken and bell pepper and sauté for 3 to 5 minutes. If mixture is drying out, add 1 to 2 tablespoons water. Add water chestnuts and stir-fry sauce and stir to combine. Cook for 1 to 2 minutes, or until vegetables and chicken are cooked through.

Red and yellow peppers are loaded with beta-carotene, an antioxidant that may protect against cancer, heart disease, and stroke.

. . . . .

Water chestnuts contain fiber, potassium, and zinc.

Per Serving
Calories 215
   Calories from Fat 70
Total Fat . . . . 8.0 g
   Saturated Fat . . . . 1.2 g
   Trans Fat . . . . 0.0 g
   Polyunsaturated Fat . . . . . . 2.4 g
   Monounsaturated Fat . . . . . . 3.5 g
Cholesterol . . . . 50 mg
Sodium . . . . 410 mg
Total Carbohydrate . . . . 15 g
   Dietary Fiber . . . . 4 g
   Sugars . . . . 6 g
Protein . . . . 22 g

GRILLED TERIYAKI CHICKEN KEBABS

Teriyaki is a favorite for all ages. Make it more interesting by skewering seasoned chicken with vegetables and fruit. Pineapple works great on the grill and echoes the sweetness of the sauce. Like a stir-fry, kebabs are a great way for vegetables to play a larger role in the main course, adding color and nutrients.

Try different teriyaki sauces to find one you like. Some are thicker with some texture; others are thinner with a soy sauce–like consistency. Garlic and ginger add brightness to the marinade, but skip them if time or ingredients are lacking.

SERVES 4 / PREP TIME: 30 MINUTES OR LESS INCLUDING MARINATING / TOTAL TIME: 45 MINUTES OR LESS

¼ cup teriyaki sauce
3 garlic cloves, minced
2 teaspoons finely chopped fresh ginger
1 cup peeled and cored pineapple, cut into 1-inch pieces, juices reserved

¾ pound boneless, skinless chicken breasts, cut into 1-inch pieces
1 red bell pepper, seeded and cut into 1-inch pieces
1 red onion, cut into 1-inch pieces

Preheat a lightly oiled grill to medium-high.

In a bowl, combine teriyaki sauce, garlic, ginger, and reserved pineapple juice. Remove and reserve 1 tablespoon of the mixture. Add chicken to bowl and marinate for 20 minutes.

Remove chicken from marinade. On skewers, thread pieces of chicken, pineapple, bell pepper, and onion.

Grill kebabs for 5 minutes, brush with reserved marinade, turn and baste again. Cook for 3 to 5 minutes, or until cooked through.

> If using wooden skewers, soak them in water while the chicken marinates to prevent them from burning. They still get a little charred, just more slowly.

Per Serving	
Calories	150
Calories from Fat	20
Total Fat	2.5 g
Saturated Fat	0.6 g
Trans Fat	0.0 g
Polyunsaturated Fat	0.6 g
Monounsaturated Fat	0.7 g
Cholesterol	50 mg
Sodium	275 mg
Total Carbohydrate	13 g
Dietary Fiber	2 g
Sugars	8 g
Protein	19 g

QUICK CHICKEN CACCIATORE

This quick-cooking version of the classic slow-braised dish is loaded with vitamin-rich bell peppers, tomatoes, garlic, and mushrooms. Using thin chicken breasts is not necessary, but dramatically speeds cooking time. Buy thin-sliced cutlets or pound thicker ones and cut them in half. Just be sure that the chicken pieces are uniform in thickness so they cook evenly.

If fresh herbs are in season, substitute them for dried, doubling the amounts and adding them at the end of cooking. Tubes of tomato paste are available at many supermarkets, making it easy to use just what is needed.

SERVES 4 / PREP TIME: 30 MINUTES OR LESS / TOTAL TIME: 1 HOUR OR LESS

¾ pound "thin sliced" or boneless, skinless chicken breasts, pounded to uniform thickness and cut in half

Salt and freshly ground black pepper

1 to 2 tablespoons all-purpose flour

2 tablespoons olive oil, divided

1 onion, halved and thinly sliced

1 red bell pepper, seeded and thinly sliced lengthwise

1 yellow bell pepper, seeded and thinly sliced lengthwise

1 (8-ounce) package mushrooms, halved if large

3 garlic cloves, minced

1 teaspoon dried basil

½ teaspoon dried oregano

½ cup dry red wine

1 (14½-ounce) can petite cut or diced tomatoes, drained

1 tablespoon tomato paste

Sprinkle the chicken with salt and pepper. Lightly coat with flour, shaking off excess.

In a large skillet over medium-high heat, add 1 tablespoon oil. Cook the chicken for 2 to 3 minutes per side. Remove the chicken and keep warm.

Add the remaining tablespoon oil. Sauté the onion, both bell peppers, and mushrooms for 8 to 10 minutes, or until softened. Add garlic, basil, and oregano and sauté for 1 minute. Add wine, tomatoes, and tomato paste and bring to a boil, stirring to combine and dislodge any bits of food that might have stuck to the bottom of the skillet. Return the chicken to the skillet, reduce the heat, cover, and simmer for 5 to 8 minutes, or until the chicken is cooked through, turning once.

Per Serving	
Calories	240
Calories from Fat	80
Total Fat	9.0 g
Saturated Fat	1.5 g
Trans Fat	0.0 g
Polyunsaturated Fat	1.4 g
Monounsaturated Fat	5.8 g
Cholesterol	50 mg
Sodium	170 mg
Total Carbohydrate	17 g
Dietary Fiber	3 g
Sugars	7 g
Protein	21 g

POACHED SALMON WITH MANGO SALSA

Poaching, a no-fat method for cooking, imparts subtle flavor while retaining moisture. This is especially critical when preparing seafood, where overcooking can dry out the fish and ruin it. Another benefit: poached fish is just as good served chilled.

Although poaching intimidates a lot of cooks, it shouldn't. No special equipment is needed, just a skillet large enough to hold the fish in a single layer with a tight-fitting lid.

This salmon can also be seared in a lightly oiled nonstick pan and topped with the salsa.

Add or substitute other fruit into the salsa, including peaches, papayas, or, for tartness, fresh cranberries.

SERVES 4 / PREP TIME: 15 MINUTES OR LESS / TOTAL TIME: 30 MINUTES OR LESS

---

2 mangoes, peeled, pitted, and chopped
¼ cup finely chopped red bell pepper
2 to 3 tablespoons fresh lime juice
2 tablespoons finely chopped red onion
2 tablespoons finely chopped fresh cilantro

1 tablespoon finely chopped jalapeño
Salt and freshly ground black pepper
2 (8-ounce) bottles of clam juice
1 lemon, sliced
1 pound salmon fillets

In a bowl, combine mangoes, bell pepper, 2 tablespoons lime juice, onion, cilantro, and jalapeño. Taste and add additional lime juice if necessary.

In a deep skillet large enough to hold the salmon in one layer, combine clam juice and lemon slices. Simmer for 5 minutes. Add the salmon, cover, and simmer for 10 minutes, or until cooked through.

Top salmon with salsa.

> Mangoes are loaded with antioxidants vitamin C and beta-carotene.
>
> . . . . .
>
> Mangoes can be a challenge to cut because they have a large, flat seed that sticks tenaciously to the fruit. Using a sharp knife, cut the fruit vertically, sliding the knife along the seed on one side. Repeat on the other side to create two large pieces. Then cut away as much of the remaining meat as you can. Remove the peel after cutting.

Per Serving	
Calories	275
Calories from Fat	90
Total Fat	10.0 g
Saturated Fat	1.8 g
Trans Fat	0.0 g
Polyunsaturated Fat	2.2 g
Monounsaturated Fat	4.8 g
Cholesterol	75 mg
Sodium	95 mg
Total Carbohydrate	22 g
Dietary Fiber	2 g
Sugars	18 g
Protein	25 g

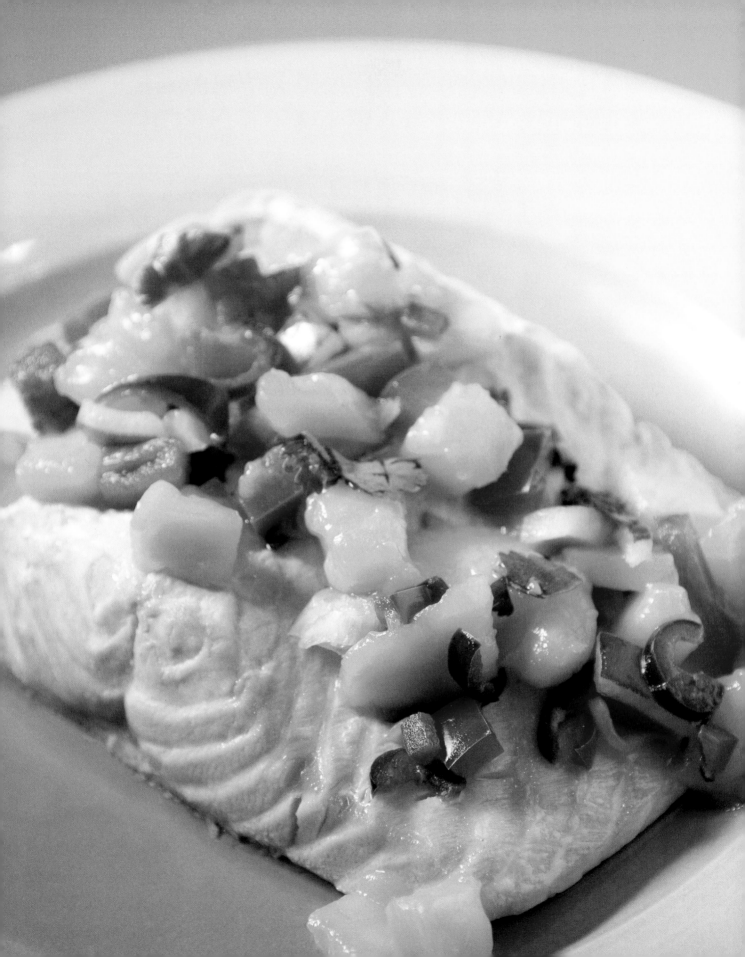

MOROCCAN SPICED CHICKEN WITH VEGETABLE COUSCOUS

Cooking your main course and side dish at the same time isn't just time efficient, it also means one less pot to wash!

Whole grain couscous has more than three times the fiber of regular couscous. Because the amount of liquid needed can vary between brands of couscous, check the box's directions for the recommended amount and adjust the recipe accordingly.

If you have green olives on hand, slice them and add with the chickpeas for added zest.

SERVES 4 / PREP TIME: 15 MINUTES OR LESS / TOTAL TIME: 45 MINUTES OR LESS

1/2 teaspoon salt
1/4 teaspoon cayenne pepper
1 teaspoon ground ginger
1 teaspoon ground cumin
1 teaspoon ground cinnamon
1 pound chicken tenders or boneless, skinless chicken breasts, pounded to uniform thickness
2 tablespoons olive oil

1/2 small red onion, finely chopped
1 carrot, finely chopped
1 garlic clove, minced
1 1/2 cups reduced–sodium chicken broth
1 cup whole wheat or regular couscous
1/2 cup canned chickpeas, rinsed and drained
2 tablespoons slivered almonds, toasted, optional

In a bowl, combine salt, cayenne pepper, ginger, cumin, and cinnamon. Coat the chicken with the spices.

In a large skillet over medium-high heat, add oil. Cook the chicken for 3 to 5 minutes per side. Remove the chicken and keep warm.

Sauté the onion, carrot, and garlic for 5 to 8 minutes, or until softened. Add broth and bring to a boil, stirring to combine. Turn off the heat, add couscous and chickpeas, and stir to combine. Return the chicken to the skillet, cover, and let stand for 5 minutes. Fluff the couscous and sprinkle with almonds.

Per Serving	
Calories	380
Calories from Fat	100
Total Fat	11.0 g
Saturated Fat	2.0 g
Trans Fat	0.0 g
Polyunsaturated Fat	2.0 g
Monounsaturated Fat	6.4 g
Cholesterol	65 mg
Sodium	590 mg
Total Carbohydrate	38 g
Dietary Fiber	5 g
Sugars	4 g
Protein	32 g

BLACK BEAN AND BUTTERNUT SQUASH CHILI

This autumnal stew is reminiscent of the bright red, orange, and golden hues of the leaves when butternut squash is in season.

Loaded with nutritious and fiber-full veggies and beans, this comforting chili fills you up without weighing you down.

SERVES 6 / PREP TIME: 30 MINUTES OR LESS / TOTAL TIME: 1 HOUR OR LESS

1 tablespoon canola oil
2 garlic cloves, minced
1 onion, chopped
1 red bell pepper, seeded and chopped
2 tablespoons chili powder
2 teaspoons ground cumin
1 teaspoon dried oregano
5 cups peeled, seeded butternut squash, cut into 1-inch pieces

1 (14½-ounce) can vegetable broth or reduced–sodium chicken broth
1 (10-ounce) can diced tomatoes with chiles, such as Ro*Tel
1 (15-ounce) can no-salt-added corn, drained
1 (15-ounce) can black beans, rinsed and drained
Salt and freshly ground black pepper

In a large stockpot over medium heat, add oil. Sauté the garlic, onion, and bell pepper for 8 to 10 minutes, or until softened. Add chili powder, cumin, and oregano and stir to combine.

Add squash, broth, and tomatoes and their juice and bring to a boil, stirring to combine. Reduce the heat, cover, and simmer for 20 minutes, stirring occasionally. Add corn and beans and simmer for 5 to 10 minutes, or until the squash is tender, stirring occasionally. Season with salt and pepper.

Per Serving	
Calories	190
Calories from Fat	35
Total Fat	4.0 g
Saturated Fat	0.4 g
Trans Fat	0.0 g
Polyunsaturated Fat	1.5 g
Monounsaturated Fat	1.8 g
Cholesterol	0 mg
Sodium	555 mg
Total Carbohydrate	35 g
Dietary Fiber	9 g
Sugars	11 g
Protein	7 g

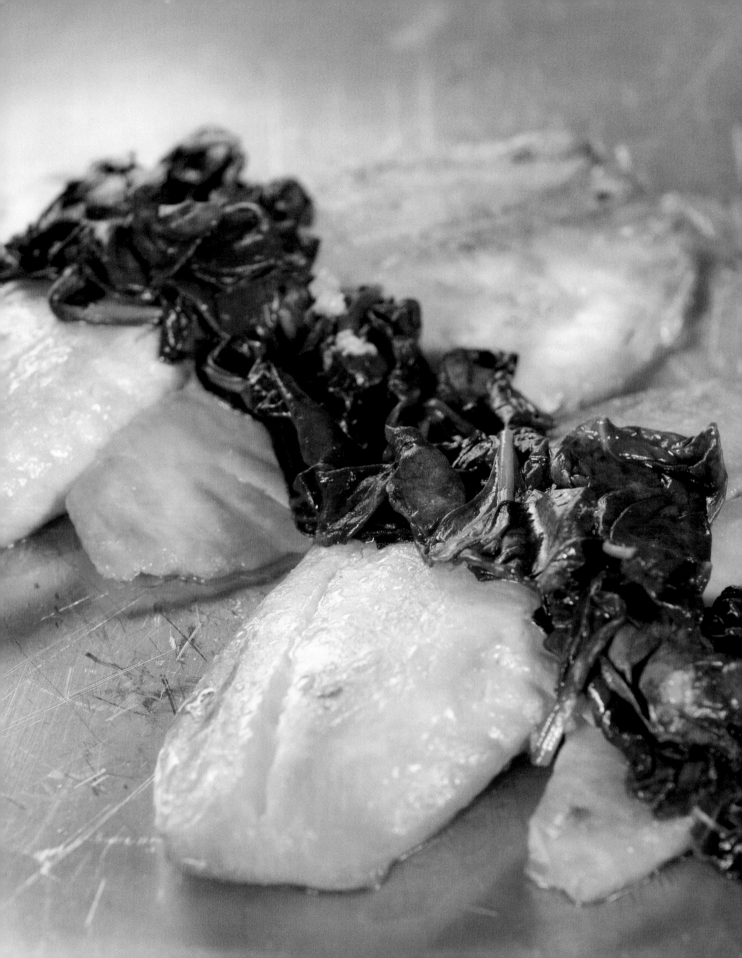

SKILLET TILAPIA WITH SAUTÉED SPINACH

This quick-cooking dish puts an ethnic spin on familiar ingredients. Tilapia is coated with a flavorful blend of Asian condiments and topped with similarly infused sautéed spinach.

Serve with brown rice.

SERVES 4 / PREP TIME: 15 MINUTES OR LESS / TOTAL TIME: 30 MINUTES OR LESS

1 tablespoon reduced–sodium soy sauce
2 teaspoons finely chopped fresh ginger
2 teaspoons rice vinegar
1 garlic clove, minced
1 teaspoon Asian sesame oil

1 pound tilapia or other thin white
 fish fillets
2 teaspoons canola oil
1 (9- or 10-ounce) bag baby spinach
1 tablespoon water

In a bowl, combine soy sauce, ginger, rice vinegar, garlic, and sesame oil. Lightly brush fish with some of the mixture.

In a large skillet, preferably nonstick, over medium-high heat, add canola oil. Add the fish and cook for 2 to 4 minutes per side, or until cooked through. Remove fish and keep warm.

Add spinach, the remaining soy mixture, and water to skillet and sauté until spinach is bright green and wilted. Push spinach to the side and return fish to skillet, cover, and cook for 30 seconds to 1 minute.

Serve fish topped with spinach.

Per Serving
Calories 155
  Calories from Fat 55
Total Fat . . . . 6.0 g
  Saturated Fat . . . . 1.4 g
  Trans Fat . . . . 0.0 g
  Polyunsaturated Fat . . . . 1.9 g
  Monounsaturated Fat . . . . . . 2.5 g
Cholesterol . . . . 75 mg
Sodium . . . . 210 mg
Total Carbohydrate . . . . 3 g
  Dietary Fiber . . . . 1 g
  Sugars . . . . 0 g
Protein . . . . 24 g

MINI MEATLOAVES

These individual meatloaves will satisfy any meat-lover, but their main components—
ground turkey breast and lean ground beef—make them much more healthful.

Line your baking sheet with aluminum foil or parchment paper to speed cleanup.

Serve with Garlic Mashed Potatoes (page 108).

SERVES 8 / PREP TIME: 15 MINUTES OR LESS / TOTAL TIME: 45 MINUTES OR LESS

¼ cup ketchup
1 tablespoon light brown sugar
½ teaspoon dry mustard
¾ pound ground turkey breast
¾ pound lean ground beef
½ cup Italian–style bread crumbs
½ (10-ounce) package frozen chopped
  spinach, thawed and drained

1 egg
1 (6-ounce) can Italian herb–seasoned
  tomato paste
2 tablespoons dried parsley
1 teaspoon Italian seasoning
1 teaspoon garlic powder
½ teaspoon salt

Preheat the oven to 350 degrees. Lightly coat a rimmed baking sheet with nonstick cooking spray.

In a bowl, combine ketchup, brown sugar, and mustard and set aside.

In a bowl, combine turkey and beef. Add bread crumbs, spinach, egg, tomato paste, parsley, Italian seasoning, garlic powder, and salt and stir gently to incorporate. Form into 8 equal-sized small loafs and place on the baking sheet.

Bake for 15 minutes, remove from the oven, and brush each loaf with ketchup mixture. Bake for 10 to 15 minutes, or until an instant-read thermometer registers 160 degrees.

Choose extra-lean ground beef to save on saturated fat and calories. Look for labels that say at least "90% lean;" you may even be able to find ground beef that is 93% or 95% lean.
. . . . .
Look for "ground turkey breast" instead of "ground turkey." If the label doesn't say "breast," you'll be getting both white and dark meat, as well as skin, in the mixture, adding a lot of saturated fat and calories.

Per Serving	
Calories	195
Calories from Fat	45
Total Fat	5 g
Saturated Fat	1.8 g
Trans Fat	0.2 g
Polyunsaturated Fat	0.5 g
Monounsaturated Fat	1.9 g
Cholesterol	80 mg
Sodium	595 mg
Total Carbohydrate	15 g
Dietary Fiber	2 g
Sugars	6 g
Protein	22 g

SAVORY SALMON AND LEEK PACKETS

These salmon fillets, perched atop a leek and spinach mixture and garnished with lemon slices and fresh dill, create an impressive main course. Wrapped in foil and baked individually, each one is like a gift for diners to unwrap and enjoy.

SERVES 4 / PREP TIME: 15 MINUTES OR LESS / TOTAL TIME: 45 MINUTES OR LESS

---

1 tablespoon olive oil
2 leeks, white and light green parts only, thinly sliced
1 (5- or 6-ounce) bag baby spinach
2 lemons

4 (4-ounce) salmon fillets, preferably skinless
Salt and freshly ground black pepper
1/4 cup white wine
1 tablespoon finely chopped fresh dill

Preheat the oven to 400 degrees.

In a large skillet over medium heat, add oil. Sauté the leeks for 5 to 7 minutes, or until softened. Add spinach and sauté until bright green and wilted.

Meanwhile, slice one lemon very thinly and squeeze 1/4 cup juice from the other lemon.

Tear off four 10-by-14-inch pieces of foil. Divide leek mixture into four parts and place in the middle of each piece of foil. Top with a piece of salmon and sprinkle with salt and pepper. Lay two to three lemon slices on top of salmon. Pull the sides of the foil up around the salmon to make a well. Drizzle each piece of salmon with 1 tablespoon wine and 1 tablespoon lemon juice. Sprinkle with dill. Fold foil around the fish, sealing well. Place the packets on a baking sheet.

Bake for 15 to 20 minutes or until cooked through. To serve, place foil packs on individual plates.

> Choose fillets of even thickness for uniform baking time.

Per Serving	
Calories	265
Calories from Fat	115
Total Fat	13.0 g
Saturated Fat	2.2 g
Trans Fat	0.0 g
Polyunsaturated Fat	2.6 g
Monounsaturated Fat	7.2 g
Cholesterol	75 mg
Sodium	90 mg
Total Carbohydrate	8 g
Dietary Fiber	1 g
Sugars	2 g
Protein	26 g

SHRIMP, BEAN, AND FETA BAKE

Serve with warm pita bread and a salad of cucumber, red onion, and Kalamata olives tossed with red wine vinaigrette.

SERVES 4 / PREP TIME: 15 MINUTES OR LESS / TOTAL TIME: 45 MINUTES OR LESS

---

1 tablespoon olive oil
1 onion, finely chopped
2 garlic cloves, minced
1 (28-ounce) can diced tomatoes, drained
1 (15½-ounce) can cannellini beans, rinsed and drained

½ cup clam juice
⅛ teaspoon cayenne pepper
1 pound large shrimp, peeled and deveined
½ cup crumbled feta cheese

Preheat the oven to 400 degrees.

In a large ovenproof skillet over medium heat, add oil. Sauté the onion for 5 to 8 minutes, or until softened. Add garlic and sauté for 1 minute. Add tomatoes, beans, clam juice, and cayenne pepper and bring to a boil, stirring to combine. Cook for 5 minutes, or until thickened, stirring frequently. Add shrimp and stir to combine. Sprinkle with the feta.

Transfer to the oven and bake for 10 minutes, or until the tomatoes are bubbly, the shrimp is cooked through, and the feta has softened. For added browning, place under the broiler for 1 to 2 minutes.

Often referred to as "white kidney beans," cannellini beans contain folate and magnesium in addition to fiber.

Per Serving	
Calories	280
Calories from Fat	80
Total Fat	9.0 g
Saturated Fat	3.5 g
Trans Fat	0.2 g
Polyunsaturated Fat	1.1 g
Monounsaturated Fat	3.5 g
Cholesterol	150 mg
Sodium	730 mg
Total Carbohydrate	27 g
Dietary Fiber	7 g
Sugars	6 g
Protein	25 g

RATATOUILLE WITH BEANS

*This hearty vegetable stew is loaded with the bounty of the summer harvest—
zucchini, eggplant, bell peppers, and fresh basil. Chickpeas add protein and texture.
Top with a sprinkle of Parmesan cheese.*

SERVES 6 / PREP TIME: 30 MINUTES OR LESS / TOTAL TIME: 1 HOUR AND 15 MINUTES OR LESS

2 tablespoons olive oil
3 garlic cloves, minced
1 onion, chopped
1 green bell pepper, seeded and
   chopped
1 red bell pepper, seeded and chopped
1 eggplant, cut into 1-inch pieces

1 zucchini, halved lengthwise and sliced
1 (28-ounce) can diced tomatoes
1 teaspoon salt
1 (15-ounce) can chickpeas, rinsed and
   drained
¼ cup thinly sliced fresh basil
⅓ cup freshly grated Parmesan cheese

In a large stockpot over medium heat, add oil. Sauté the garlic, onion, and both bell peppers for 8 to 10 minutes, or until softened. Add eggplant and zucchini and cook for 8 to 10 minutes, stirring frequently.

Add tomatoes and their juice and stir to combine. Reduce the heat to low, cover, and cook for 30 minutes, or until the vegetables are tender, stirring occasionally. Add chickpeas and basil and stir to combine. Cook for 1 minute.

Top individual servings with cheese.

Tomatoes are a virtual powerhouse of nutrients,
rich in lycopene, vitamins A and C, folate,
potassium, and fiber.

Per Serving	
Calories	215
Calories from Fat	70
Total Fat	8.0 g
Saturated Fat	1.7 g
Trans Fat	0.0 g
Polyunsaturated Fat	1.3 g
Monounsaturated Fat	4.1 g
Cholesterol	5 mg
Sodium	765 mg
Total Carbohydrate	32 g
Dietary Fiber	8 g
Sugars	13 g
Protein	9 g

SALMON IN ASIAN BROTH

This elegant dish layers flavors and textures with stunning results. Sautéed spinach is topped with steamed salmon and surrounded by a soy-sherry-ginger broth. A garnish of scallions and toasted sesame seeds completes the presentation.

Even though three things are going at once, the dish comes together in about 15 minutes.

SERVES 2 / PREP TIME: 15 MINUTES OR LESS / TOTAL TIME: 30 MINUTES OR LESS

---

3 tablespoons plus 1 teaspoon reduced–sodium soy sauce
3 tablespoons dry sherry
3 tablespoons water
1 tablespoon finely julienned fresh ginger plus additional for garnish
2 teaspoons granulated sugar

1 teaspoon Asian sesame oil
1 (5- or 6-ounce) bag baby spinach
2 (4-ounce) salmon fillets, preferably skinless
1 scallion, thinly sliced
1 teaspoon sesame seeds, toasted

In a saucepan, combine soy sauce, sherry, water, ginger, and sugar and bring to a boil. Cover and keep warm over very low heat.

Lightly coat a steamer basket with nonstick cooking spray. Set the basket in a large stockpot with water filled to just below the basket. Add salmon. Place over medium-high heat, cover, and cook for 6 to 8 minutes, or until cooked through. Do not overcook.

While salmon is cooking, in a skillet over medium-high heat, add sesame oil. Sauté the spinach until bright green and wilted.

Divide spinach in two large soup bowls. If necessary, remove skin from salmon. Place fish on top of spinach. Pour soy broth over fish and sprinkle with scallions, sesame seeds, and additional ginger, if desired.

Salmon, in addition to being low in saturated fat, provides protein, heart-healthy omega-3 fatty acids, and B vitamins. Some studies show omega-3 fatty acids are linked to improved mental function.

. . . . .

Toasting sesame seeds adds a nutty flavor. Cook them in a dry skillet until fragrant and golden, shaking frequently to prevent burning.

Per Serving
Calories 295
  Calories from Fat 115
Total Fat . . . . 13.0 g
  Saturated Fat . . . . 2.2 g
  Trans Fat . . . . 0.0 g
  Polyunsaturated Fat . . . . 3.5 g
  Monounsaturated Fat . . . . . . 5.9 g
Cholesterol . . . . 75 mg
Sodium . . . . 1065 mg
Total Carbohydrate . . . . 12 g
  Dietary Fiber . . . . 2 g
  Sugars . . . . 7 g
Protein . . . . 29 g

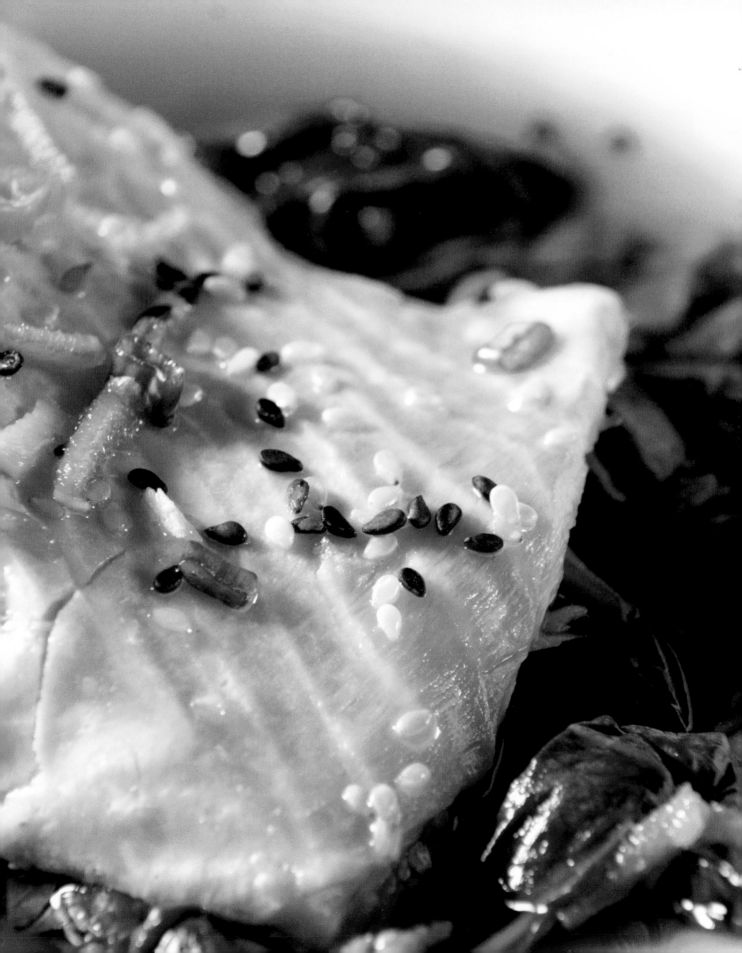

FIG, GINGER, AND BUTTERNUT SQUASH RISOTTO

Risotto demands a lot of vigilance because the slow absorption of broth is key to the creamy, yet firm, quality of the finished dish. But it's definitely worth the effort. Although this is a rich-tasting dish, it actually has very little fat.

SERVES 4 TO 6 / PREP TIME: 15 MINUTES OR LESS / TOTAL TIME: 1 HOUR AND 15 MINUTES OR LESS

4 to 5 cups reduced–sodium chicken broth, divided
5 dried figs, stems removed
1 tablespoon olive oil
1/4 cup finely chopped onion
1 tablespoon finely chopped fresh ginger

2 cups peeled, seeded, and finely chopped butternut squash (about 12 ounces)
1 1/2 cups Arborio or Carnaroli rice
1 cup dry white wine
1/2 cup freshly grated Parmesan cheese
Salt and freshly ground black pepper

In a saucepan, combine 1 cup chicken broth and figs and bring to a simmer. With a slotted spoon, transfer the figs to a cutting board, finely chop, and set aside. Add the remaining 4 cups chicken broth to the pan and bring to a light simmer. Cover and keep warm over very low heat.

In a large saucepan or stockpot over medium heat, add oil. Sauté the onion, ginger, and squash for 5 to 8 minutes, or until softened. Add rice and sauté for 1 minute. Add wine and stir until almost completely absorbed.

Begin slowly adding the broth, 1/2 cup at a time, stirring frequently. Wait until each addition is almost completely absorbed before adding more, 3 to 5 minutes for each addition. Continue to add broth, stirring frequently, for 30 to 40 minutes, or until the risotto has a creamy texture but is still slightly firm to the bite. You might not need to use all of the liquid.

Stir figs and cheese into the risotto. Season with salt and pepper and serve immediately.

Dried fruits make great snacks and healthy additions to salads, side dishes, and even main courses.

· · · · ·

Unlike regular rice, risotto should be served a bit runny, with the rice still slightly firm in the center.

Per Serving (for 4 servings)
Calories 425
   Calories from Fat 70
Total Fat . . . . 8.0 g
   Saturated Fat . . . . 2.7 g
   Trans Fat . . . . 0.0 g
   Polyunsaturated Fat . . . . 0.8 g
   Monounsaturated Fat . . . . . . 3.9 g
Cholesterol . . . . 10 mg
Sodium . . . . 595 mg
Total Carbohydrate . . . . 75 g
   Dietary Fiber . . . . 4 g
   Sugars . . . . 15 g
Protein . . . . 13 g

MEXICAN "LASAGNA"

This casserole layers a piquant tomato sauce with tortillas, beans, and corn, putting a healthier twist on the classic chilaquiles casserole. It is best made with slightly stale tortillas; if possible, leave them out for a couple of hours to dry out before assembling the dish.

While most chilaquiles are loaded with fat, this one includes just enough cheese to make the dish rich and satisfying without going overboard.

SERVES 6 TO 8 / PREP TIME: 15 MINUTES OR LESS / TOTAL TIME: 45 MINUTES OR LESS

7 (6-inch) corn tortillas
2 (14½-ounce) cans Mexican-style stewed tomatoes
1 cup fresh cilantro
1 (15-ounce) can no-salt-added corn, drained

1 (15-ounce) can black beans, rinsed and drained
1½ cups "Mexican-style" shredded cheese

Preheat the oven to 375 degrees.

Leave three tortillas whole, cut three into halves, and cut one into quarters. Set aside.

In a food processor, pulse the tomatoes and cilantro to combine. Drain of excess liquid.

In a bowl, combine corn and black beans.

In an 8-by-8-inch baking pan, spread ½ cup of tomato mixture over the bottom of the dish. Cover with one whole tortilla, two tortilla halves and one quarter to fit the pan. Top with half of the bean mixture, 1 cup of tomato mixture, and ½ cup cheese. Cover the sauce with tortillas arranged as before. Top with the remaining beans, 1 cup of tomato mixture, and ½ cup of cheese. Cover with the remaining tortillas (there will be one extra quarter). Top with 1 cup tomato mixture and the remaining cheese.

Cover with foil and bake for 15 to 20 minutes. Uncover and bake for 10 to 15 minutes, or until the cheese melts and the casserole is heated through.

Canned vegetables can be a good alternative to fresh vegetables, but look for low-sodium or "no-salt-added" varieties.

Per Serving (for 6 servings)	
Calories	280
Calories from Fat	90
Total Fat	10.0 g
Saturated Fat	5.3 g
Trans Fat	0.0 g
Polyunsaturated Fat	1.1 g
Monounsaturated Fat	2.7 g
Cholesterol	30 mg
Sodium	620 mg
Total Carbohydrate	37 g
Dietary Fiber	9 g
Sugars	11 g
Protein	14 g

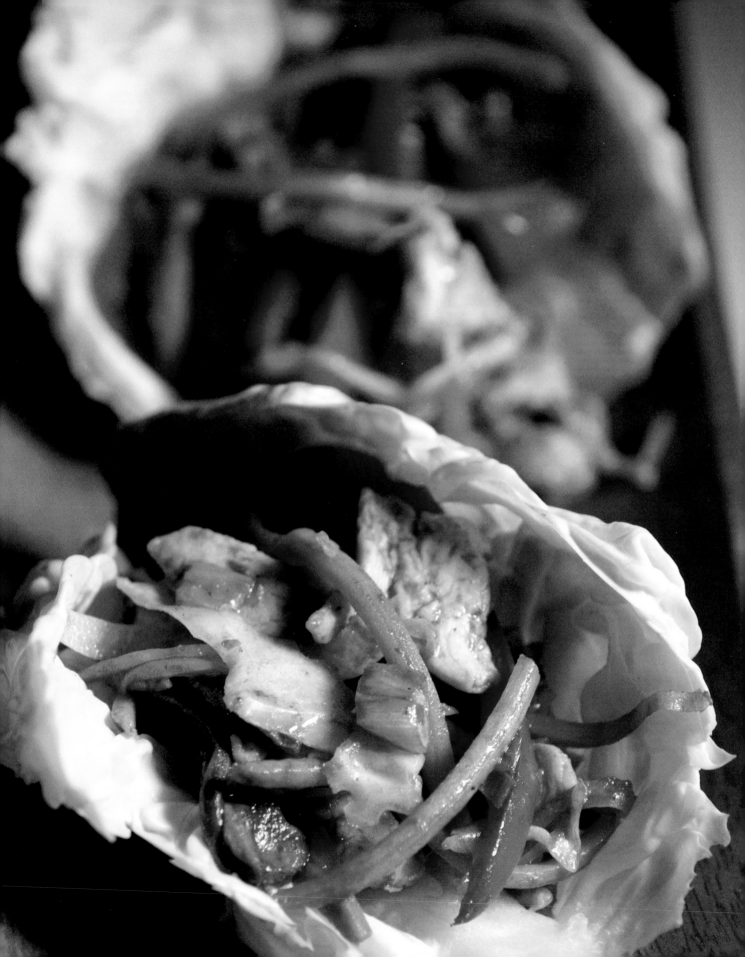

MOO SHU CHICKEN LETTUCE WRAPS

Making moo shu at home is a breeze and more healthful when you use lettuce leaves as wrappers instead of the traditional Chinese flour pancakes. Just spoon the chicken mixture into the lettuce "cups."

This dish can also be made with beef, shrimp, or pork. Shiitake or other wild mushrooms can be substituted as well.

SERVES 4 / PREP TIME: 15 MINUTES OR LESS / TOTAL TIME: 30 MINUTES OR LESS

1 tablespoon canola oil
2 cups sliced mushrooms
3/4 pound boneless, skinless chicken
   breasts, cut into very thin strips
3 cups shredded cabbage or coleslaw mix
1/2 cup matchstick-cut carrots

1/2 cup thinly sliced red bell pepper
2 scallions, thinly sliced
3 tablespoons hoisin sauce, or to taste
1 small head Boston or Bibb lettuce,
   leaves separated and core discarded

In a wok or large skillet over high heat, add oil. Sauté the mushrooms for 1 to 2 minutes. Add chicken, cabbage, carrots, bell pepper, and scallions and sauté for 5 to 7 minutes, or until tender. Add hoisin sauce and stir to combine. Cook for 1 to 2 minutes, or until vegetables and chicken are cooked through. If sauce is too thick, add 1 tablespoon water.

Spoon moo shu into lettuce leaves. Top with a small dollop of hoisin, if desired.

Leftover cabbage mix can be used to make Caraway Cole Slaw (page 107).

Per Serving
Calories 185
  Calories from Fat 55
Total Fat . . . . 6.0 g
  Saturated Fat . . . . 0.9 g
  Trans Fat . . . . 0.0 g
  Polyunsaturated Fat . . . . . . 1.8 g
  Monounsaturated Fat . . . . . . 2.9 g
Cholesterol . . . . 50 mg
Sodium . . . . 230 mg
Total Carbohydrate . . . . 12 g
  Dietary Fiber . . . . 3 g
  Sugars . . . . 7 g
Protein . . . . 21 g

FETTUCCINE WITH TOMATO–HERB SAUCE

This no-cook sauce has the vibrancy of a pesto,
but without added fat from nuts or cheese. The oil has been scaled back,
and tomatoes, either canned or fresh, balance the herbs.

Inspired by chef Mario Batali and the Italian salsa verde—a green sauce made with
capers and herbs—this dish is fresh and flavorful, but does not require a lot of effort.

SERVES 6 / PREP TIME: 15 MINUTES OR LESS / TOTAL TIME: 30 MINUTES OR LESS

12 ounces fettuccine
½ cup fresh mint, packed
½ cup fresh basil, packed
½ cup fresh Italian parsley, packed
¼ cup capers, drained
3 tablespoons extra–virgin olive oil

1 (15-ounce) can whole tomatoes,
   drained, or 2 ripe medium plum
   tomatoes
1 garlic clove, peeled
1 teaspoon crushed red pepper flakes
1 teaspoon freshly ground black pepper
¼ teaspoon salt

Prepare fettuccine according to package directions for al dente (just firm). Reserve ¼ cup pasta water and drain.

Meanwhile, in a blender or food processor, while pasta is cooking, purée mint, basil, parsley, capers, tomatoes, garlic, red pepper flakes, black pepper, and oil to form a smooth paste.

In a serving bowl, combine pasta and sauce. If sauce is too thick, dilute with pasta water, 1 tablespoon at a time.

Although some cooks may consider parsley as just a garnish, it actually provides antioxidant protection and is rich in vitamins A, C, and K, and folate.
. . . . .
Heart-healthy olive oil contains monounsaturated fat and is rich in polyphenols—phytochemicals that may provide several health benefits. Extra-virgin olive oil contains more polyphenols than regular olive oil.

Per Serving	
Calories	310
Calories from Fat	70
Total Fat	8.0 g
Saturated Fat	1.2 g
Trans Fat	0.0 g
Polyunsaturated Fat	1.2 g
Monounsaturated Fat	5.2 g
Cholesterol	0 mg
Sodium	285 mg
Total Carbohydrate	49 g
Dietary Fiber	4 g
Sugars	2 g
Protein	10 g

STIR-FRIED PORK, GREEN BEANS, AND SHIITAKE MUSHROOMS

A stir-fry is a great way to incorporate vegetables into your meal, allowing them to shine as star ingredients while the protein takes a supporting role. Feel free to mix and match veggies and protein to suit your taste. Oyster sauce adds richness to the dish.

SERVES 4 / PREP TIME: 15 MINUTES OR LESS / TOTAL TIME: 30 MINUTES OR LESS

1 tablespoon canola oil

¼ cup chopped onion

3 garlic cloves, minced

¼ teaspoon crushed red pepper flakes, or to taste

¾ pound green beans, trimmed and sliced into 1½-inch pieces

1 red bell pepper, seeded and thinly sliced

¾ pound boneless pork loin chop(s), visible fat removed and cut into very thin strips

8 ounces shiitake mushrooms, stemmed and sliced

¼ cup oyster sauce

In a wok or large skillet over high heat, add oil. Sauté the onion, garlic, and red pepper flakes for 1 minute. Add green beans and bell pepper and sauté for 3 to 5 minutes. Add pork and mushrooms and sauté for 3 to 5 minutes. If mixture is drying out, add 1 to 2 tablespoons water. Add oyster sauce and stir to combine. Cook for 1 to 2 minutes, or until vegetables and pork are cooked through.

Red bell peppers provide vitamin A, vitamin C, and folate.

Per Serving	
Calories	210
Calories from Fat	80
Total Fat	9.0 g
Saturated Fat	2.2 g
Trans Fat	0.0 g
Polyunsaturated Fat	1.6 g
Monounsaturated Fat	4.5 g
Cholesterol	45 mg
Sodium	450 mg
Total Carbohydrate	14 g
Dietary Fiber	4 g
Sugars	4 g
Protein	19 g

STUFFED GREEK CHICKEN BREASTS

Imagine cutting into a chicken breast and finding a delectable surprise—a savory spinach and feta cheese filling. Suddenly, a plain chicken breast is something special.

Depending on the shape of the chicken breasts, you might not use all the filling. You can also use Sautéed Spinach with Garlic (page 125) as a filling.

Just add rice and a salad and dinner is ready.

SERVES 4 / PREP TIME: 15 MINUTES OR LESS / TOTAL TIME: 45 MINUTES OR LESS

1 (10-ounce) package frozen chopped spinach, thawed and drained
1/4 cup feta cheese
Grated zest of 1 lemon
4 teaspoons Greek seasoning
Salt and freshly ground black pepper
4 (4-ounce) boneless, skinless chicken breasts
1 tablespoon canola oil

Preheat the oven to 350 degrees.

In a bowl, combine spinach, feta, and lemon zest.

Using a paring knife, cut a pocket in the side of the thickest part of the breast, a bit more than halfway through the width and length of the breast. Make sure not to poke through the meat. Stuff the breast with spinach mixture. Use a toothpick or wooden skewer to close the flap.

Lightly coat chicken with Greek seasoning and sprinkle with salt and pepper.

In a large ovenproof skillet over medium-high heat, add oil. Cook chicken for 3 to 5 minutes per side.

Transfer to the oven and bake for 8 to 12 minutes, or until cooked through.

Coating chicken with a seasoning blend is simple and delivers a lot of oomph. Greek seasoning—a blend of onion, garlic, spearmint, and oregano—is a great complement to the dish.

Per Serving	
Calories	205
Calories from Fat	80
Total Fat	9.0 g
Saturated Fat	2.5 g
Trans Fat	0.1 g
Polyunsaturated Fat	1.8 g
Monounsaturated Fat	3.5 g
Cholesterol	75 mg
Sodium	215 mg
Total Carbohydrate	4 g
Dietary Fiber	2 g
Sugars	1 g
Protein	28 g

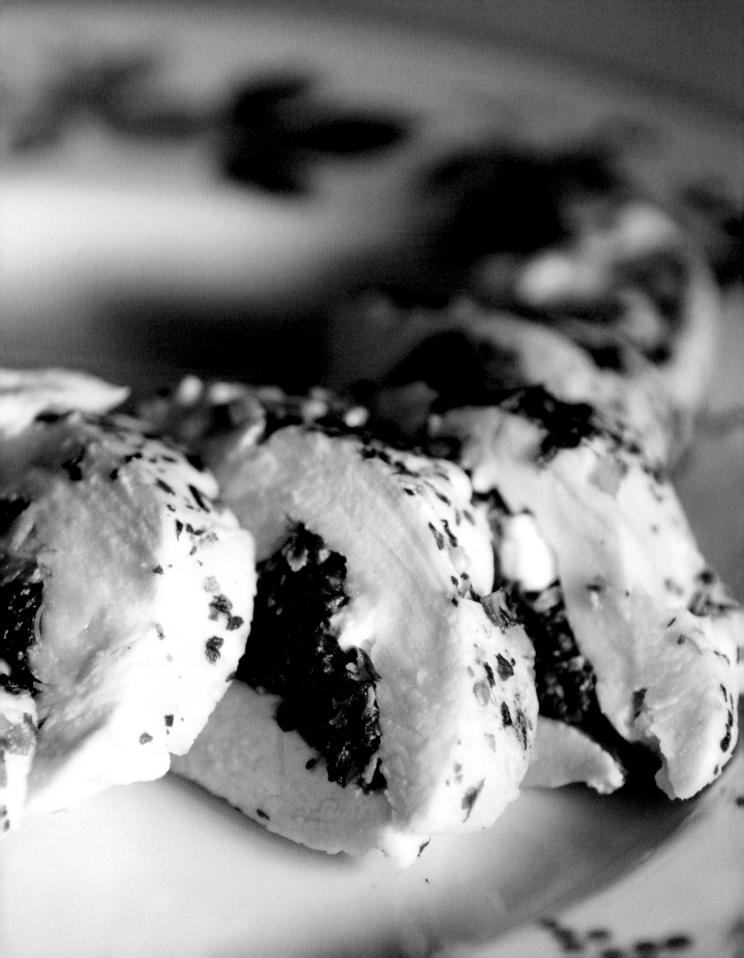

SEAFOOD STEW

This delicious blend of tomatoes, seafood, and aromatics is easy enough for a quick dinner, but elegant enough to impress guests. Choose the seafood that looks freshest at the fish counter. For a more dramatic presentation, add clams or mussels.

SERVES 4 TO 6 / PREP TIME: 15 MINUTES OR LESS / TOTAL TIME: 45 MINUTES OR LESS

1 tablespoon olive oil
2 garlic cloves, minced
1 onion, chopped
1 celery stalk, chopped
1 green bell pepper, seeded and
   chopped

1 (28-ounce) can diced tomatoes
2 (8-ounce) bottles clam juice
3/4 pound white fish (such as cod or
   tilapia), cut into pieces
1/2 pound shrimp, peeled and deveined
16 clams or mussels, optional

In a stockpot over medium heat, add oil. Sauté the garlic, onion, celery, and green pepper for 5 to 8 minutes, or until softened.

Add tomatoes and clam juice and bring to a boil, stirring to combine. Reduce the heat and simmer for 10 to 15 minutes, stirring occasionally. Add the fish and cook for 3 to 4 minutes. Add the shrimp and clams and cook for 3 to 5 minutes, or until shrimp is cooked through and clams open, stirring occasionally. Discard any clams that do not open.

Many supermarkets now sell containers of prechopped "trinity mix"—a combination of onion, celery, and bell peppers. Buy a tub to save on prep time.

Per Serving (for 4 servings)
Calories 200
  Calories from Fat 40
Total Fat . . . . 4.5 g
  Saturated Fat . . . . 0.7 g
  Trans Fat . . . . 0.0 g
  Polyunsaturated Fat . . . . 0.9 g
  Monounsaturated Fat . . . . . . 2.7 g
Cholesterol . . . . 105 mg
Sodium . . . . 775 mg
Total Carbohydrate . . . . 15 g
  Dietary Fiber . . . . 3 g
  Sugars . . . . 9 g
Protein . . . . 25 g

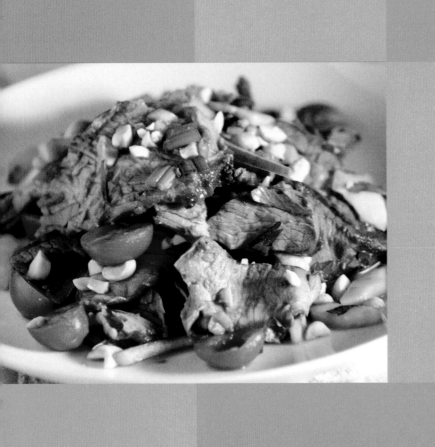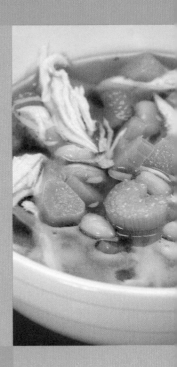

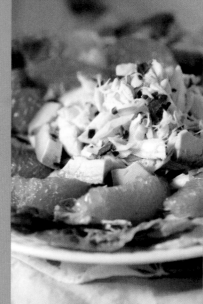

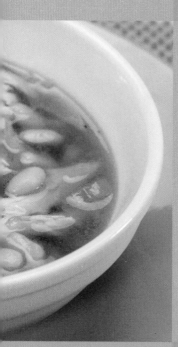

SOUPS, SALADS, AND SANDWICHES

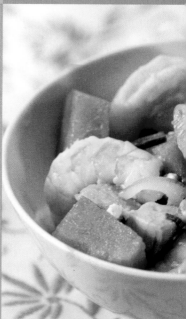

Refreshing. Elegant. Hearty. Exotic. No matter what you're in the mood for, we've got you covered. Our soups, salads, and sandwiches creatively combine ingredients both unique and usual, providing delightful twists that are sure to satisfy. Pair a comforting bowl of soup or a trendy roll-up with a tasty salad, and nourish your body with these delicious treats.

SOUTHWEST CHICKEN TORTILLA SOUP

This tomato-based soup, loaded with chicken, corn, and just enough spice to make it interesting, is topped with crunchy homemade tortilla strips.

For a less textured soup, break up the tomatoes with your hands, a knife, or a food processor before adding them to the soup.

If you have some chopped cilantro on hand, sprinkle it on individual portions just before serving.

SERVES 4 / PREP TIME: 15 MINUTES OR LESS / TOTAL TIME: 45 MINUTES OR LESS

---

1 tablespoon canola oil
1 onion, chopped
1 garlic clove, minced
1/2 teaspoon chili powder
1/8 teaspoon cayenne pepper, or to taste
4 cups reduced–sodium chicken broth
1 (14 1/2-ounce) can Mexican-style stewed tomatoes

1/2 pound boneless, skinless chicken breasts, cut into 1/2-inch pieces
1 cup fresh, frozen, or canned no-salt-added corn, drained
3 scallions, thinly sliced
2 tablespoons fresh lime juice
1 (6-inch) corn tortilla, sliced into thin strips

In a large stockpot over medium heat, add oil. Sauté the onion for 5 to 8 minutes, or until softened. Add garlic, chili powder, and cayenne pepper and sauté for 1 minute.

Add broth and tomatoes and their juice and bring to a boil, stirring to combine and to break up the tomatoes. Reduce the heat, cover, and simmer for 10 to 15 minutes, stirring occasionally. Add chicken and corn and simmer for 5 minutes. Add scallions and lime juice and cook for 1 minute, or until the chicken is cooked through.

Meanwhile, preheat the oven to 300 degrees. Place the tortilla strips on a baking sheet and bake for 12 to 15 minutes, or until crispy, stirring and checking every 3 to 5 minutes.

Top soup with tortilla strips.

Per Serving	
Calories	205
Calories from Fat	55
Total Fat	6.0 g
Saturated Fat	0.8 g
Trans Fat	0.0 g
Polyunsaturated Fat	1.8 g
Monounsaturated Fat	2.8 g
Cholesterol	35 mg
Sodium	770 mg
Total Carbohydrate	21 g
Dietary Fiber	5 g
Sugars	11 g
Protein	17 g

AROMATIC BUTTERNUT SQUASH AND APPLE SOUP

The best offerings of fall are used to create
this highly aromatic, creamy soup.

SERVES 6 / PREP TIME: 30 MINUTES OR LESS / TOTAL TIME: 1 HOUR OR LESS

1 tablespoon canola oil
1 onion, chopped
½ teaspoon ground cinnamon
½ teaspoon ground cardamom
¼ teaspoon ground nutmeg
7 cups peeled, seeded, and coarsely chopped butternut squash (about 1 medium squash)

3 Granny Smith apples, peeled, cored, and chopped
1 tablespoon finely chopped fresh ginger
3 cups reduced–sodium chicken broth or vegetable broth
1 cup apple cider or juice
Salt and freshly ground black pepper

In a large stockpot over medium heat, add oil. Sauté the onion for 5 to 8 minutes, or until softened. Add cinnamon, cardamom, and nutmeg and stir to combine. Add squash, apples, and ginger and sauté for 1 minute.

Add broth and bring to a boil, stirring to combine. Reduce the heat, cover, and simmer for 20 to 30 minutes, or until the squash is very tender, stirring occasionally.

Cool slightly and purée the soup in a food processor or blender in batches, only filling the processing bowl halfway. Return soup to stockpot and add apple cider. Stir to combine and heat through. Season with salt and pepper.

Per Serving	
Calories	150
Calories from Fat	25
Total Fat	3.0 g
Saturated Fat	0.2 g
Trans Fat	0.0 g
Polyunsaturated Fat	0.8 g
Monounsaturated Fat	1.4 g
Cholesterol	0 mg
Sodium	260 mg
Total Carbohydrate	32 g
Dietary Fiber	3 g
Sugars	17 g
Protein	3 g

BLACK BEAN SOUP WITH CILANTRO CREAM

Hearty black bean soup gets an upscale makeover with a swirl of cilantro cream.
Using canned beans cuts hours off the prep time for this classic soup.

SERVES 4 / PREP TIME: 30 MINUTES OR LESS / TOTAL TIME: 1 HOUR OR LESS

½ cup fresh cilantro
¼ cup reduced–fat or regular sour
   cream
1 tablespoon low-fat (1%) or skim milk
1 tablespoon canola oil
2 garlic cloves, minced
1 onion, chopped
1 carrot, chopped

1 celery stalk, chopped
1 jalapeño, seeded and finely chopped
2 teaspoons ground cumin
2 (15-ounce) cans black beans, rinsed
   and drained
4 cups reduced–sodium chicken broth
   or vegetable broth
Salt and freshly ground black pepper

In a food processor with the motor running, purée cilantro. Add sour cream and milk. Set aside.

In a stockpot over medium heat, add oil. Sauté the garlic, onion, carrot, celery, and jalapeño for 8 to 10 minutes, or until softened. Add cumin and sauté for 30 seconds. Add black beans and stir to combine.

Add broth and bring to a boil, stirring to combine. Reduce the heat and simmer for 20 to 30 minutes, stirring occasionally.

In a food processor, purée 3 cups of soup and add back into the pot, or use an immersion blender to purée directly in the pot. Season with salt and pepper.

Pour soup into individual bowls and swirl in 1 tablespoon of the cilantro-cream mixture.

Per Serving	
Calories	260
Calories from Fat	45
Total Fat	5 g
Saturated Fat	1.2 g
Trans Fat	0.0 g
Polyunsaturated Fat	1.5 g
Monounsaturated Fat	2.4 g
Cholesterol	5 mg
Sodium	695 mg
Total Carbohydrate	39 g
Dietary Fiber	12 g
Sugars	8 g
Protein	15 g

SUPER VEGGIE SOUP

This soup is loaded with veggies, beans, and pasta to keep you satisfied.

Make this soup a staple in summer when gardens are overflowing with zucchini, spinach, and beans, or use it when you have lots of leftover veggies in your fridge. Let your imagination run wild—add whatever is plentiful to make it your own!

SERVES 8 / PREP TIME: 30 MINUTES OR LESS / TOTAL TIME: 45 MINUTES OR LESS

2 tablespoons olive oil

2 large or 3 small leeks, white part only, thinly sliced

1 carrot, sliced

1 celery stalk, sliced

1 small zucchini, halved lengthwise and sliced

8 cups reduced–sodium chicken broth or vegetable broth

1 (28-ounce) can diced tomatoes

1 tablespoon dried oregano

1 tablespoon dried basil

Salt and freshly ground black pepper

½ cup small pasta shapes or orzo

1 cup green beans, trimmed and cut into 1-inch pieces

1 cup spinach

1 cup canned cannellini or navy beans, rinsed and drained

½ cup freshly grated Parmesan cheese, optional

In a stockpot over medium heat, add oil. Sauté the leeks for 8 to 10 minutes, or until softened. Add carrots, celery, and zucchini and cook for 5 to 8 minutes, or until softened, stirring occasionally.

Add broth, tomatoes and their juice, oregano, and basil. Sprinkle with salt and pepper and bring to a boil, stirring to combine. Add pasta. Reduce the heat and simmer for 5 minutes, stirring occasionally. Add green beans, spinach, and cannellini beans and simmer for 5 minutes, stirring occasionally.

Top individual servings with cheese.

Leeks have a tendency to have a lot of dirt near the root end. Before using, make sure to clean them well.

Per Serving
Calories 165
    Calories from Fat 35
Total Fat . . . . 4.0 g
    Saturated Fat . . . . 0.5 g
    Trans Fat . . . . 0.0 g
    Polyunsaturated Fat . . . . 0.7 g
    Monounsaturated Fat . . . . . . 2.5 g
Cholesterol . . . . 0 mg
Sodium . . . . 740 mg
Total Carbohydrate . . . . 26 g
    Dietary Fiber . . . . 5 g
    Sugars . . . . 7 g
Protein . . . . 8 g

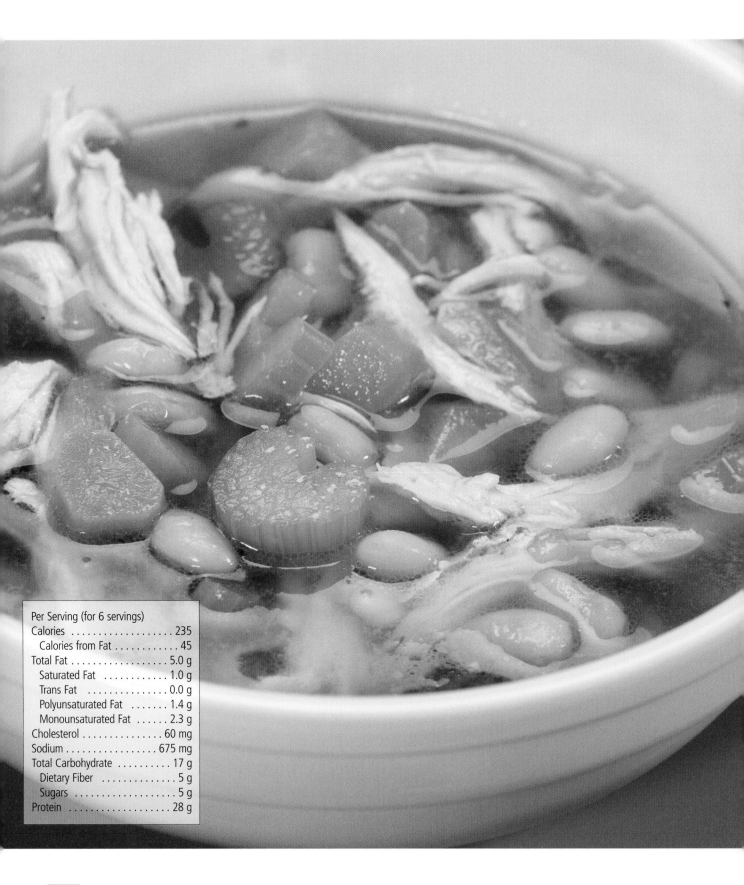

Per Serving (for 6 servings)

Calories 235
  Calories from Fat 45
Total Fat . . . . 5.0 g
  Saturated Fat . . . . 1.0 g
  Trans Fat . . . . 0.0 g
  Polyunsaturated Fat . . . . 1.4 g
  Monounsaturated Fat . . . . . . 2.3 g
Cholesterol . . . . 60 mg
Sodium . . . . 675 mg
Total Carbohydrate . . . . 17 g
  Dietary Fiber . . . . 5 g
  Sugars . . . . 5 g
Protein . . . . 28 g

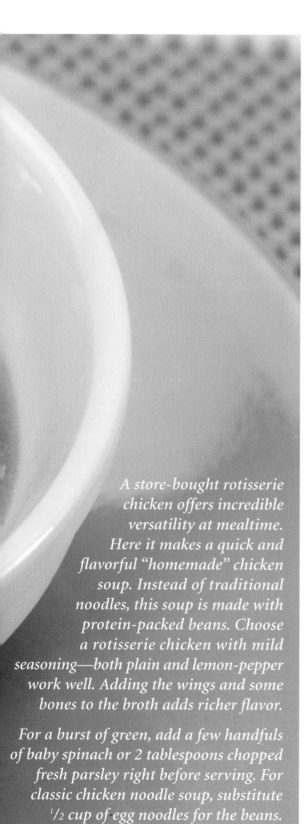

A store-bought rotisserie chicken offers incredible versatility at mealtime. Here it makes a quick and flavorful "homemade" chicken soup. Instead of traditional noodles, this soup is made with protein-packed beans. Choose a rotisserie chicken with mild seasoning—both plain and lemon-pepper work well. Adding the wings and some bones to the broth adds richer flavor.

For a burst of green, add a few handfuls of baby spinach or 2 tablespoons chopped fresh parsley right before serving. For classic chicken noodle soup, substitute $^{1}/_{2}$ cup of egg noodles for the beans.

CHICKEN AND WHITE BEAN SOUP

SERVES 6 TO 8 / PREP TIME: 15 MINUTES OR LESS
TOTAL TIME: 1 HOUR OR LESS

---

1 rotisserie chicken breast section or 3 cups chopped white chicken meat
1 tablespoon canola oil
3 carrots, sliced
2 celery stalks, sliced
1 onion, chopped
2 cups water
6 cups reduced–sodium chicken broth
1 (15-ounce) can Great Northern beans, rinsed and drained
Salt and freshly ground black pepper

Remove wings from chicken and reserve. Remove skin from breast and discard. Shred the meat from the breast and break off breastbones.

In a stockpot over medium heat, add oil. Sauté the carrots, celery, onion, chicken wings, and breastbones for 8 to 10 minutes, or until vegetables soften.

Add water and chicken broth and bring to a boil, stirring to combine. Reduce the heat, cover, and simmer for 15 to 20 minutes. Add beans and chicken meat and cook for 5 minutes. If too thick, add additional broth or water. Discard bones and wings before serving. Season with salt and pepper.

Store-bought rotisserie chicken can be a lifesaver on those busy nights. Add it to salads, soups, sandwiches, or quesadillas.

RED CLAM CHOWDER

Reminiscent of Manhattan–style clam chowder, this tomato-based soup skips the bacon and substitutes lots of clams and Old Bay Seasoning blend for a burst of flavor. If you use a food processor to purée the tomatoes, use it to prep the vegetables too. Use the pulse button to chop the onion, celery, and potato. Do each vegetable separately.

SERVES 4 / PREP TIME: 15 MINUTES OR LESS / TOTAL TIME: 1 HOUR AND 15 MINUTES OR LESS

1 (28-ounce) can whole tomatoes
1 tablespoon olive oil
1 onion, finely chopped
2 celery stalks, finely chopped
1 small potato, peeled and finely chopped

3 garlic cloves, minced
2 (8-ounce) bottles clam juice
1 tablespoon Old Bay Seasoning
4 (6½-ounce) cans chopped clams in juice
Salt and freshly ground black pepper

In a blender or food processor, purée the tomatoes and their juice until smooth.

In a stockpot over medium heat, add oil. Sauté the onion, celery, and potato for 8 to 10 minutes, or until softened. Add garlic and Old Bay and sauté for 1 minute.

Add tomatoes and clam juice and bring to a boil, stirring to combine and to dislodge any bits of food that might have stuck to the bottom of the pot. Reduce the heat, cover, and simmer for 30 to 40 minutes, or until the potatoes have softened, stirring occasionally. Add clams and their juices and simmer for 5 to 10 minutes, stirring occasionally. Season with salt and pepper.

Celery has a surprising amount of potassium and compounds called phthalides, both of which have been linked to reduced blood pressure. Store celery in a tub of ice water in the fridge so it stays crunchy.

Per Serving	
Calories	175
Calories from Fat	40
Total Fat	4.5 g
Saturated Fat	0.6 g
Trans Fat	0.0 g
Polyunsaturated Fat	0.9 g
Monounsaturated Fat	2.5 g
Cholesterol	35 mg
Sodium	1220 mg
Total Carbohydrate	21 g
Dietary Fiber	3 g
Sugars	10 g
Protein	14 g

MUSHROOM–BARLEY SOUP

*First cultivated in ancient Egypt, barley dates back to between 6000 and 5000 BC.
Once a popular offering to the gods, barley was found alongside
other "treasures" in the tomb of King Tut.*

*Use a variety of mushrooms, such as shiitakes and baby portobellos,
for added flavor and texture. Quick-cooking barley speeds things up.
If using pearl barley, allow about 20 minutes additional cooking time.*

Barley will continue to absorb liquid upon standing so, if necessary, add broth.

SERVES 6 / PREP TIME: 15 MINUTES OR LESS / TOTAL TIME: 1 HOUR OR LESS

---

2 tablespoons canola oil

3 carrots, chopped

3 garlic cloves, minced

2 celery stalks, chopped

1 onion, chopped

1 red bell pepper, seeded and chopped

6 cups sliced mushrooms (any variety)

8 cups reduced–sodium chicken broth
  or vegetable broth

1 cup quick-cooking or pearl barley

1 tablespoon reduced–sodium soy sauce

In a large stockpot over medium-high heat, add oil. Sauté the carrots, garlic, celery, onion, and bell pepper for 8 to 10 minutes, or until softened. Add mushrooms and sauté for 5 to 8 minutes, or until they give off most of their liquid.

Add broth and bring to a boil, stirring to combine. Add barley and stir to combine. Reduce the heat and simmer for 15 to 20 minutes, or until the barley is tender and the soup thickens, stirring occasionally. Stir in the soy sauce.

Cremini mushrooms, a younger version of portobellos, offer B vitamins, potassium, protein, folate, and fiber, with only 30 to 40 calories per half cup.

Per Serving	
Calories	210
Calories from Fat	55
Total Fat	6.0 g
Saturated Fat	0.4 g
Trans Fat	0.0 g
Polyunsaturated Fat	2.2 g
Monounsaturated Fat	3.1 g
Cholesterol	0 mg
Sodium	808 mg
Total Carbohydrate	35 g
Dietary Fiber	6 g
Sugars	9 g
Protein	5 g

LENTIL–VEGETABLE SOUP

Lentils date back to the ancient Greeks and Romans.

If you like a thicker soup, purée 3 cups of soup in a food processor and add back into the pot, or use an immersion blender to purée directly in the pot.

SERVES 8 / PREP TIME: 15 MINUTES OR LESS / TOTAL TIME: 1 HOUR OR LESS

1 tablespoon olive oil
1 onion, chopped
2 carrots, chopped
2 celery stalks, chopped
8 cups reduced–sodium chicken broth
  or vegetable broth
1 (28-ounce) can diced tomatoes

1⅓ cups dried lentils
4 tablespoons chopped fresh Italian
  parsley, divided
1 teaspoon dried thyme
1 cup dry white or red wine, optional
Salt and freshly ground black pepper

In a large stockpot over medium heat, add oil. Sauté the onions, carrots, and celery for 8 to 10 minutes, or until softened.

Add broth, tomatoes and their juice, lentils, 2 tablespoons parsley, and thyme and bring to a boil, stirring to combine. Reduce the heat, cover, and simmer for 20 to 25 minutes, or until the lentils are tender, stirring occasionally.

Add wine and cook for 5 minutes. Season with salt and pepper and add the remaining 2 tablespoons parsley.

Unlike many legumes, lentils don't need to be soaked before using and cook in less than a half hour. In addition to protein, lentils contain potassium and iron.

Per Serving	
Calories	170
Calories from Fat	20
Total Fat	2.5 g
Saturated Fat	0.3 g
Trans Fat	0.0 g
Polyunsaturated Fat	0.5 g
Monounsaturated Fat	1.3 g
Cholesterol	0 mg
Sodium	725 mg
Total Carbohydrate	28 g
Dietary Fiber	9 g
Sugars	7 g
Protein	12 g

ROASTED ROOT VEGETABLE SOUP

Making roasted vegetable soup couldn't be easier. Spread the veggies out on a baking sheet, stick them in the oven until soft and lightly caramelized, and then purée with broth. No standing vigil over the stockpot, constantly stirring for even cooking.

Line your baking sheet with aluminum foil or parchment paper to speed cleanup.

SERVES 6 / PREP TIME: 30 MINUTES OR LESS / TOTAL TIME: 1 HOUR AND 15 MINUTES OR LESS

1 pound carrots, peeled and cut into
1½-inch pieces
1 pound parsnips, peeled and cut into
1½-inch pieces
1 sweet potato, peeled and cut into
1½-inch pieces

2 tablespoons chopped fresh ginger
2 tablespoons olive oil
2 tablespoons honey
Salt and freshly ground black pepper
6 cups reduced–sodium chicken broth
or vegetable broth, heated

Preheat the oven to 400 degrees.

On a rimmed baking sheet, combine carrots, parsnips, sweet potato, and ginger. Drizzle with oil and honey and toss to lightly coat. Sprinkle with salt and pepper.

Roast for 40 to 50 minutes, or until tender and slightly charred, stirring every 10 to 15 minutes for even roasting.

Transfer vegetables to a food processor or blender, add 1 to 2 cups broth, and blend until smooth. Transfer to a stockpot, adding the remaining broth to achieve desired consistency, and heat through.

Root vegetables—like carrots, parsnips, beets, and turnips—are just plain good for you. Packed with vitamins and minerals, they typically keep well in the refrigerator for 1 to 2 weeks.

Per Serving	
Calories	180
Calories from Fat	45
Total Fat	5.0 g
Saturated Fat	0.6 g
Trans Fat	0.0 g
Polyunsaturated Fat	0.9 g
Monounsaturated Fat	3.6 g
Cholesterol	0 mg
Sodium	560 mg
Total Carbohydrate	32 g
Dietary Fiber	5 g
Sugars	16 g
Protein	2 g

TUNA MELT

This classic sandwich balances indulgence and nutritious eating. Tuna, a pantry staple, is enriched with chopped veggies to make it more filling and to add vitamins.

Try it on whole wheat bread, or hollow out a half bagel and fill the "moat" with the mixture before sprinkling on cheese. Heat in a toaster oven or place under the broiler.

SERVES 3 / PREP TIME: 15 MINUTES OR LESS / TOTAL TIME: 30 MINUTES OR LESS

---

1 (6-ounce) can white tuna packed in water, drained

1/4 red bell pepper, chopped

1 celery stalk, halved lengthwise and sliced

1 small carrot, chopped, or 1/4 cup matchstick-cut carrots, chopped

1 tablespoon good-quality light mayonnaise, such as Hellmann's

2 teaspoons Dijon mustard

Salt and freshly ground black pepper

3 slices whole wheat bread

1 tomato, sliced

1/4 cup shredded cheddar cheese

In a bowl, flake tuna. Add celery, carrot, bell pepper, mayonnaise, and mustard and stir to combine. Season with salt and pepper. Divide mixture on bread, top with tomato slices, and sprinkle with cheese.

Position an oven rack 4 to 6 inches from the heat and preheat the broiler.

Place sandwiches on a baking sheet and broil until cheese melts.

Using tuna packed in water instead of oil is an easy way to save on calories, and with all the flavors in this dish, you won't even miss the oil!

Per Serving

Calories	205
Calories from Fat	65
Total Fat	7.0 g
Saturated Fat	2.6 g
Trans Fat	0.0 g
Polyunsaturated Fat	1.5 g
Monounsaturated Fat	1.9 g
Cholesterol	25 mg
Sodium	530 mg
Total Carbohydrate	19 g
Dietary Fiber	4 g
Sugars	4 g
Protein	19 g

BARBECUE CHICKEN QUESADILLA

A chicken quesadilla is a great way to use up the remnants of a purchased rotisserie chicken or leftovers from last night's chicken dinner. Tossing the meat in barbecue sauce creates a fusion of two cuisines, giving a classic an unexpected twist.

In the mood for something more traditional? No problem. Skip the barbecue sauce and serve with salsa.

SERVES 1 / PREP TIME: 15 MINUTES OR LESS / TOTAL TIME: 15 MINUTES OR LESS

½ cup chopped cooked chicken
1 tablespoon barbecue sauce
2 (8-inch) whole wheat tortillas

½ cup shredded reduced-fat cheddar
  or "Mexican-style" shredded cheese
2 tablespoons chopped fresh cilantro
1 tablespoon finely chopped red onion

In a bowl, combine chicken and barbecue sauce.

Lightly coat a skillet with nonstick cooking spray. Place one tortilla in the skillet and sprinkle with cheese, chicken, cilantro, and onion. Top with the remaining tortilla. Cook over medium heat until the bottom tortilla is golden and cheese begins to melt. Flip and finish cooking.

Per Serving	
Calories	565
Calories from Fat	200
Total Fat	22.0 g
Saturated Fat	8.9 g
Trans Fat	0.0 g
Polyunsaturated Fat	3.6 g
Monounsaturated Fat	7.3 g
Cholesterol	100 mg
Sodium	1280 mg
Total Carbohydrate	48 g
Dietary Fiber	6 g
Sugars	8 g
Protein	41 g

CRAB SALAD WITH GRAPEFRUIT, AVOCADO, AND BABY GREENS

This is a wonderful "ladies who lunch" salad. Sections of pink grapefruit and wedges of lush avocado surround a mound of lightly dressed crabmeat. It couldn't be more "taste-full."

SERVES 2 / PREP TIME: 30 MINUTES OR LESS / TOTAL TIME: 30 MINUTES OR LESS

---

1 pink or ruby red grapefruit
2 tablespoons extra–virgin olive oil
1 tablespoon fresh lemon juice
1/4 teaspoon granulated sugar
1/2 pound fresh crabmeat, picked over for cartilage
2 tablespoons chopped fresh Italian parsley

1 tablespoon chopped fresh chives plus additional for garnish
Salt and freshly ground black pepper
1/2 avocado, sliced
4 cups (or 6.5-ounce bag) cut baby Bibb or Boston lettuce

Peel and segment grapefruit over a bowl to catch juice. Reserve 1 tablespoon juice and grapefruit pieces separately.

In a bowl, combine oil, lemon juice, sugar, and reserved grapefruit juice.

In a bowl, combine crabmeat, parsley, and chives. Add 1 1/2 tablespoons dressing and toss to combine. Season with salt and pepper.

Combine lettuce with the remaining dressing. Divide on individual plates. Add a scoop of crabmeat salad and surround with grapefruit segments and avocado slices.

Grapefruit is not only loaded with vitamin C, but red varieties also contain the antioxidant lycopene.

. . . . .

To easily section the grapefruit, use a paring knife to cut the top and bottom so it can sit upright. Cut off the rind and pith in long downward slices. Carefully cut the sections free, following the natural guide of the fruit.

Per Serving	
Calories	345
Calories from Fat	180
Total Fat	20.0 g
Saturated Fat	2.8 g
Trans Fat	0.0 g
Polyunsaturated Fat	2.5 g
Monounsaturated Fat	13.9 g
Cholesterol	65 mg
Sodium	360 mg
Total Carbohydrate	21 g
Dietary Fiber	5 g
Sugars	11 g
Protein	23 g

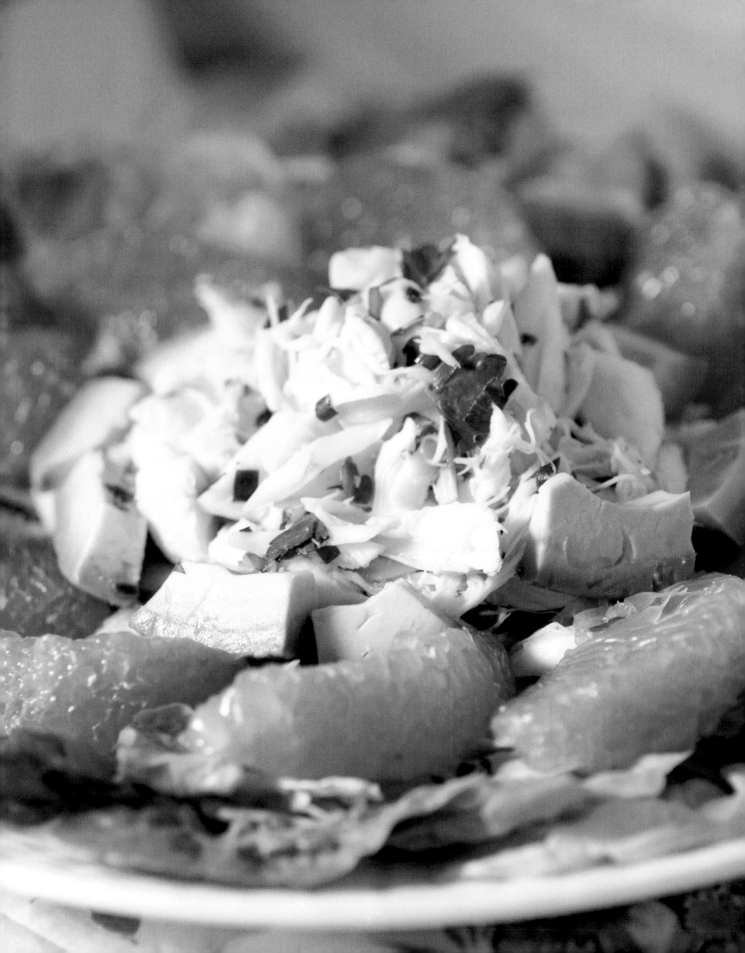

EGGS-TRAORDINARY TACO

A vegetable omelet is an unexpected filling inside a warm tortilla coated with melted cheese and salsa. It's a quick, satisfying hot meal, great for breakfast, lunch, or dinner.

Use a 10-inch nonstick skillet with sloped sides for the omelet. The base of the pan should be 8 inches, exactly the right size for the tortilla.

Don't worry if your omelet doesn't flip perfectly. If you have a hard time flipping it, slide it onto a plate and then place it back in the pan, uncooked side down.

Feel free to add your own embellishments. Try adding sautéed spinach or chopped ham, mushrooms, or tomatoes.

SERVES 1 / PREP TIME: 15 MINUTES OR LESS / TOTAL TIME: 15 MINUTES OR LESS

---

2 eggs
1 scallion, thinly sliced
¼ cup chopped green bell pepper

2 tablespoons shredded reduced-fat cheddar or "Mexican-style" shredded cheese
1 (8-inch) whole wheat tortilla
2 tablespoons salsa

In a bowl, beat eggs. Add scallion and bell pepper and stir to combine.

Coat a 10-inch skillet, preferably nonstick, with nonstick cooking spray. Over medium heat, add egg mixture and cook without stirring for 30 seconds to 1 minute, or until the eggs are almost set on the bottom. Continue cooking, using a spatula to lift the edges of the egg toward the center of the skillet, while gently tilting the pan so the uncooked eggs run underneath the bottom of the omelet, without stirring, until almost set. With a spatula, turn over to finish cooking.

Meanwhile, sprinkle the cheese over the tortilla and microwave for 20 to 30 seconds, or until the cheese melts. Cover tortilla with salsa. Use a spatula to place eggs onto the tortilla. Fold tortilla over the eggs and eat like a taco.

Per Serving	
Calories	325
Calories from Fat	145
Total Fat	16.0 g
Saturated Fat	5.2 g
Trans Fat	0.0 g
Polyunsaturated Fat	2.5 g
Monounsaturated Fat	5.7 g
Cholesterol	435 mg
Sodium	740 mg
Total Carbohydrate	25 g
Dietary Fiber	4 g
Sugars	4 g
Protein	20 g

CURRIED CHICKEN SALAD

Chicken salad goes international with a combination of curry powder and bottled chutney. The addition of fresh and dried fruits adds flavor and fiber.

Serve on bread or in a whole wheat pita for a sensational sandwich, or spoon atop mixed greens for a memorable salad.

SERVES 8 / PREP TIME: 30 MINUTES OR LESS / TOTAL TIME: 30 MINUTES OR LESS

---

1 pound boneless, skinless chicken breasts
¼ cup good-quality light mayonnaise, such as Hellmann's
¼ cup nonfat plain yogurt
¼ cup Major Grey's chutney
1 tablespoon curry powder, or to taste
1 apple, chopped

¼ cup currants, raisins, or golden raisins
¼ cup chopped dried apricots
1 celery stalk, chopped
1 scallion, thinly sliced, optional
Salt and freshly ground black pepper
3 tablespoons chopped peanuts or toasted slivered almonds, optional

Lightly coat a steamer basket with nonstick cooking spray. Set the basket in a large stockpot with water filled to just below the basket. Add chicken in a single layer, place over medium heat, cover, and cook for 10 to 12 minutes, or until cooked through. Do not overcook. Set aside to cool. When cool enough to handle, shred or chop.

Meanwhile, in a bowl, combine mayonnaise, yogurt, chutney, and curry powder. Add chicken, apple, currants, apricots, celery, and scallion and stir to combine. Season with salt and pepper. Sprinkle with nuts just before serving.

Per Serving	
Calories	165
Calories from Fat	35
Total Fat	4.0 g
Saturated Fat	0.8 g
Trans Fat	0.0 g
Polyunsaturated Fat	1.7 g
Monounsaturated Fat	1.1 g
Cholesterol	35 mg
Sodium	190 mg
Total Carbohydrate	18 g
Dietary Fiber	1 g
Sugars	13 g
Protein	14 g

SPICY SOBA SALAD

Soba are long, thin noodles made from buckwheat. They cook quickly and have a mild, nutty flavor that pairs nicely with tahini, a paste made from ground sesame seeds. Ginger, crushed red pepper flakes, and jalapeño give this salad a little kick while keeping sodium levels reasonable.

To save time, prepare the vegetables and the dressing while the noodles cook.

SERVES 6 / PREP TIME: 15 MINUTES OR LESS / TOTAL TIME: 30 MINUTES OR LESS

½ pound buckwheat noodles (soba)
½ cup reduced–sodium chicken broth
  or vegetable broth
2 tablespoons tahini
2 tablespoons cider or rice vinegar
1 tablespoon reduced–sodium soy sauce
½ teaspoon crushed red pepper flakes
½-inch piece fresh ginger, peeled
1 garlic clove, peeled
Freshly ground black pepper

1 cup (packed) mung bean sprouts
1 cucumber, peeled, seeded, and cut
  into long, thin strips
½ red bell pepper, halved lengthwise,
  seeded, and cut into long, thin strips
1 jalapeño, seeded and finely chopped,
  optional
¼ cup chopped roasted peanuts
Lettuce leaves
¼ cup chopped fresh cilantro

Prepare noodles according to package directions for al dente (just firm). Drain, rinse with cold water, and drain again. Set aside.

In a blender or food processor, combine broth, tahini, vinegar, soy sauce, red pepper flakes, ginger, and garlic and blend until smooth. Season with pepper.

Meanwhile, in a bowl, combine bean sprouts, cucumber, bell pepper, jalapeño, peanuts, and noodles. Toss with enough dressing to coat. Serve over lettuce leaves and garnish with chopped cilantro.

Per Serving	
Calories	185
Calories from Fat	55
Total Fat	6 g
Saturated Fat	0.8 g
Trans Fat	0.0 g
Polyunsaturated Fat	2.2 g
Monounsaturated Fat	2.5 g
Cholesterol	0 mg
Sodium	255 mg
Total Carbohydrate	27 g
Dietary Fiber	3 g
Sugars	3 g
Protein	9 g

MEDITERRANEAN CHICKEN SALAD

In this main course salad, grilled chicken is layered on a bed of greens dotted with chewy dried fruit, crunchy pine nuts, and creamy goat cheese (also known as chèvre).

If using cooked "thin sliced" chicken breasts, lay them whole on top of the salad, or slice regular boneless chicken breasts. If time is of the essence, use white meat from a store-bought rotisserie chicken.

SERVES 4 / PREP TIME: 15 MINUTES OR LESS / TOTAL TIME: 30 MINUTES OR LESS

¼ cup extra–virgin olive oil
2 tablespoons balsamic vinegar
2 teaspoons Dijon mustard
½ teaspoon granulated sugar
¼ teaspoon salt
½ pound "thin sliced" or regular boneless, skinless chicken breasts
8 cups loosely packed "European" lettuce mix or other assorted lettuce mix

1 cucumber, peeled, seeded, and chopped
½ cup dried and sweetened cranberries, such as Craisins
2 tablespoons finely chopped chives
¼ cup pine nuts, toasted
4 ounces goat cheese, crumbled

Preheat a lightly oiled grill to medium-high.

In a bowl, combine oil, vinegar, mustard, sugar, and salt and stir well to combine. Remove 2 tablespoons and brush chicken with that dressing.

Grill chicken for 2 to 3 minutes per side for thin cutlets, 5 to 7 minutes per side for regular breasts, or until cooked through. Remove from grill and let rest for 5 minutes before slicing.

In a bowl, combine lettuce, cucumber, cranberries, and chives. Add enough dressing to lightly coat. Divide on individual plates. Top with chicken, pine nuts, and goat cheese.

Per Serving	
Calories	375
Calories from Fat	225
Total Fat	25 g
Saturated Fat	6.5 g
Trans Fat	0.0 g
Polyunsaturated Fat	4.6 g
Monounsaturated Fat	12.1 g
Cholesterol	45 mg
Sodium	325 mg
Total Carbohydrate	20 g
Dietary Fiber	2 g
Sugars	15 g
Protein	20 g

When using olive oil for salad dressings or applications aside from cooking oil, it's worth choosing extra–virgin olive oil. This fruitier, more flavorful oil is made from the first cold pressing of the olives and has the lowest acidity level.

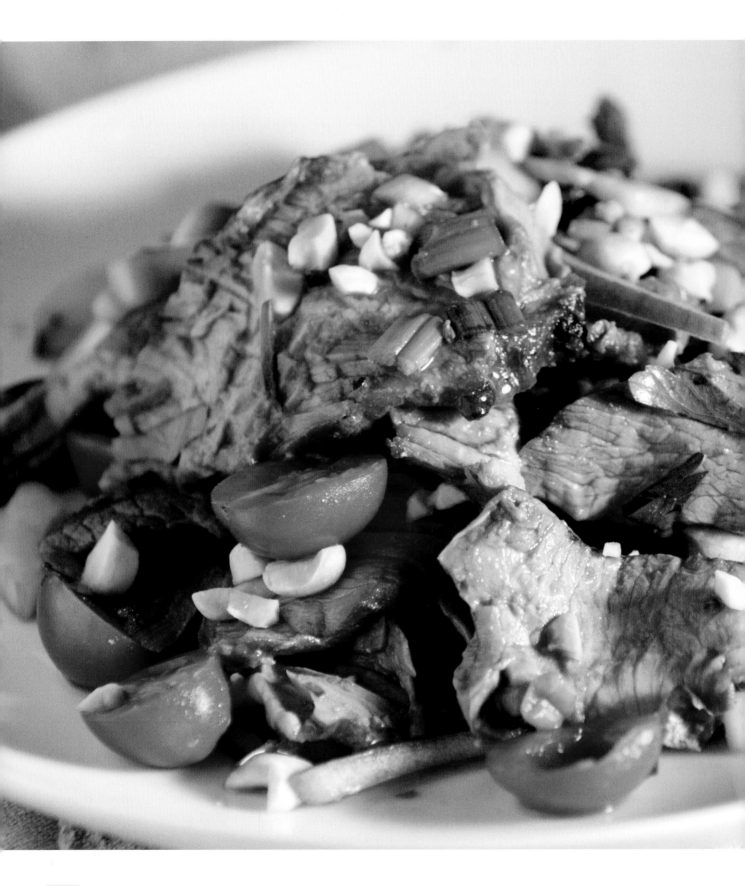

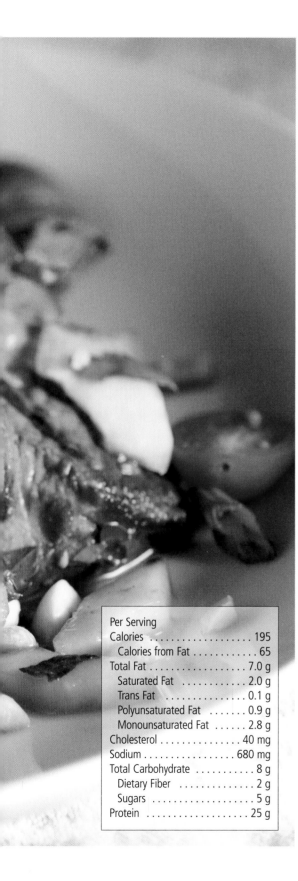

ASIAN BEEF SALAD

Get to know the ingredients in the international foods aisle of your supermarket. You can have a culinary world tour without leaving your backyard. The chili paste (also known as Sambal Oelek) used in this recipe provides just enough heat to make things interesting.

This spicy salad can also be made with chicken or shrimp.

SERVES 4 / PREP TIME: 15 MINUTES OR LESS
TOTAL TIME: 30 MINUTES OR LESS

1 pound sirloin steak, trimmed of excess fat
3 tablespoons fresh lime juice
1 tablespoon fish sauce
1 tablespoon reduced–sodium soy sauce
1 teaspoon granulated sugar
$\frac{1}{2}$ teaspoon chili paste, chili and garlic sauce, or crushed
  red pepper flakes, or to taste
1 cucumber, peeled, seeded, quartered lengthwise, and
  thinly sliced
$\frac{1}{4}$ red onion, thinly sliced
1 cup halved grape tomatoes
2 tablespoons chopped fresh cilantro
2 tablespoons chopped fresh mint
2 scallions, thinly sliced
2 tablespoons chopped roasted peanuts

Preheat a lightly oiled grill to medium-high.

Grill steak for 7 to 10 minutes per side for medium-rare. Remove from grill and let rest for 5 minutes before slicing into thin strips.

Meanwhile, in a serving bowl, combine lime juice, fish sauce, soy sauce, sugar, and chili paste.

Add steak and toss to coat. Add cucumber, onion, tomatoes, cilantro, mint, and scallions and gently toss to combine. Sprinkle with peanuts.

Per Serving	
Calories	195
Calories from Fat	65
Total Fat	7.0 g
Saturated Fat	2.0 g
Trans Fat	0.1 g
Polyunsaturated Fat	0.9 g
Monounsaturated Fat	2.8 g
Cholesterol	40 mg
Sodium	680 mg
Total Carbohydrate	8 g
Dietary Fiber	2 g
Sugars	5 g
Protein	25 g

TOMATOES STUFFED WITH SHRIMP SALAD

During the summer months, nothing beats a big, juicy, ripe tomato. Not only are they delicious on their own or as part of a side salad, tomatoes are the ideal edible "container" for a cool seafood salad made with tuna, crabmeat, salmon, or shrimp.

Using precooked shrimp from the supermarket seafood department makes this a great last-minute meal.

SERVES 2 / PREP TIME: 15 MINUTES OR LESS / TOTAL TIME: 15 MINUTES OR LESS

½ pound cooked peeled and deveined shrimp, chopped
2 tablespoons finely chopped celery
1 tablespoon good-quality light mayonnaise, such as Hellmann's
1 tablespoon thinly sliced chives

2 teaspoons chopped fresh dill
1 tablespoon capers, drained and chopped
Salt and freshly ground black pepper
2 large ripe tomatoes

In a bowl, combine shrimp, celery, mayonnaise, chives, dill, and capers. Season with salt and pepper.

Remove tops and core of tomatoes. Scoop out insides, discarding the seeds but keeping the flesh. Chop flesh and place in bowl with shrimp. Stir to combine. Divide mixture between tomatoes.

Per Serving	
Calories	170
Calories from Fat	35
Total Fat	4.0 g
Saturated Fat	0.8 g
Trans Fat	0.0 g
Polyunsaturated Fat	2.0 g
Monounsaturated Fat	0.9 g
Cholesterol	225 mg
Sodium	455 mg
Total Carbohydrate	8 g
Dietary Fiber	2 g
Sugars	5 g
Protein	25 g

TUNA–BEAN SALAD

Tuna and canned beans are a protein-packed combo.
It you want, serve over a bed of baby spinach or other greens.

SERVES 6 / PREP TIME: 30 MINUTES OR LESS / TOTAL TIME: 30 MINUTES OR LESS

2 (6-ounce) cans white tuna packed in water, drained

1 (15-ounce) can Cannellini beans, rinsed and drained

2 plum tomatoes, cut into ½-inch pieces

1 red bell pepper, seeded and cut into ½-inch pieces

1 (14-ounce) can artichoke hearts packed in water, drained and quartered

1 cup fresh green beans, blanched and cut into 1-inch pieces

½ cup chopped carrots or bagged matchstick-cut carrots, chopped

½ cup sliced Kalamata olives, optional

¼ cup chopped red onion

¼ cup chopped fresh Italian parsley

¼ cup fresh lemon juice

2 tablespoons extra–virgin olive oil

Salt and freshly ground black pepper

In a bowl, flake tuna. Add beans, tomatoes, bell pepper, artichoke hearts, green beans, carrots, olives, onion, and parsley and stir to combine. Drizzle with lemon juice and oil and gently toss to combine. Season with salt and pepper.

Per Serving
Calories 200
  Calories from Fat 55
Total Fat . . . . 6.0 g
  Saturated Fat . . . . 0.8 g
  Trans Fat . . . . 0.0 g
  Polyunsaturated Fat . . . . 1.0 g
  Monounsaturated Fat . . . . . . 3.5 g
Cholesterol . . . . 15 mg
Sodium . . . . 350 mg
Total Carbohydrate . . . . 20 g
  Dietary Fiber . . . . 6 g
  Sugars . . . . 3 g
Protein . . . . 19 g

TURKEY BURGERS WITH CRANBERRY CHUTNEY

Think of these burgers as a taste of Thanksgiving—with a twist.
The savory chutney, flavored with mustard seeds, ginger, and crushed red pepper
flakes, makes a piquant relish. Keep a bag or two of cranberries in your freezer
to make this—and other tasty dishes—throughout the year.

Serve as is or on whole wheat buns. Burgers can also be grilled.

SERVES 4 / PREP TIME: 15 MINUTES OR LESS / TOTAL TIME: 30 MINUTES OR LESS

1/4 cup light brown sugar	1/4 teaspoon salt
3 tablespoons cider vinegar	1/4 teaspoon crushed red pepper flakes
4 tablespoons finely chopped onion, divided	1 cup fresh cranberries
1 garlic clove, minced	1 egg
1 tablespoon finely chopped fresh ginger	1 pound ground turkey breast
1/2 teaspoon mustard seeds	1 tablespoon Dijon mustard
	2 tablespoons plain bread crumbs

In a saucepan over medium-high heat, combine brown sugar, vinegar, 2 tablespoons onion, mustard seeds, garlic, ginger, salt, and red pepper flakes and bring to a boil. Reduce heat and simmer for 3 to 5 minutes. Add cranberries and simmer until berry skins start to split, stirring occasionally. Continue cooking until syrup thickens, 3 to 5 minutes. Set aside to cool. It will become firmer upon standing.

In a bowl, beat egg. Add turkey, the remaining 2 tablespoons onion, mustard, and bread crumbs, gently stirring to combine. Form into four patties.

Coat a large skillet with nonstick cooking spray. Over medium-high heat, cook burgers for 5 to 7 minutes per side, or until an instant-read thermometer registers 165 degrees. If burgers are thick (more than an inch), cover skillet for the last 5 minutes of cooking.

Top burgers with a dollop of cranberry chutney.

> Cranberries contain antioxidants and other phytonutrients that may help protect against heart disease, cancer, and other diseases. They also contain proanthocyanidins, which may help prevent and treat urinary tract infections.

Per Serving	
Calories	230
Calories from Fat	20
Total Fat	2.5 g
Saturated Fat	0.7 g
Trans Fat	0.0 g
Polyunsaturated Fat	0.5 g
Monounsaturated Fat	0.8 g
Cholesterol	125 mg
Sodium	330 mg
Total Carbohydrate	21 g
Dietary Fiber	2 g
Sugars	16 g
Protein	29 g

GREEK CHICKEN AND TZATZIKI PITAS

Packaged "thin sliced" chicken breasts are now available at most supermarkets. These cutlets cook in a jiffy and fit snugly in a pita pocket for lunch or a light dinner. If they aren't available, slice regular breasts lengthwise to make even, easy to grill cutlets.

Tzatziki is a yogurt and cucumber-based sauce. To add a little zing, chop up some pepperoncini and Kalamata olives and add to sauce.

SERVES 4 / PREP TIME: 30 MINUTES OR LESS / TOTAL TIME: 30 MINUTES OR LESS

1 tablespoon olive oil
1 tablespoon plus 1 teaspoon lemon juice, divided
3 garlic cloves, minced, divided
1 teaspoon dried oregano
4 "thin sliced" boneless, skinless chicken breasts or 2 boneless, skinless chicken breasts, sliced lengthwise
1 (6-ounce) container nonfat plain yogurt

½ cucumber, peeled, seeded, and chopped
2 to 3 shakes hot sauce, such as Tabasco, or to taste
1 tablespoon chopped fresh dill
Fresh lemon juice
Salt and freshly ground black pepper
4 lettuce leaves
1 tomato, sliced
2 (6- to 7-inch) whole wheat pitas, halved

In a shallow plate, combine oil, 1 tablespoon lemon juice, 2 minced garlic cloves, and oregano. Add chicken, turning to coat, and marinate for 15 minutes.

In a bowl, combine yogurt, cucumber, hot sauce, dill, and the remaining garlic and 1 teaspoon lemon juice. Season with salt and pepper.

Preheat a lightly oiled grill to medium-high.

Remove chicken from marinade and sprinkle with salt and pepper. Grill chicken for 2 to 3 minutes per side, or until cooked through.

Divide lettuce and tomato in pita halves. Add chicken and top with sauce.

Per Serving	
Calories	250
Calories from Fat	55
Total Fat	6.0 g
Saturated Fat	1.2 g
Trans Fat	0.0 g
Polyunsaturated Fat	1.2 g
Monounsaturated Fat	2.8 g
Cholesterol	70 mg
Sodium	160 mg
Total Carbohydrate	21 g
Dietary Fiber	2 g
Sugars	5 g
Protein	30 g

SOUTHWESTERN BEAN BURGERS

These pillowy vegetarian burgers are a welcome change from standard fare and are so much better for you. Tuck them in a whole wheat bun or serve as is with a dollop of salsa.

Prep the carrots by using a food processor fit with a shredding blade (the blade with the smaller holes if there are two) and then switch to the main chopping blade to mash the beans.

SERVES 6 / PREP TIME: 15 MINUTES OR LESS / TOTAL TIME: 30 MINUTES OR LESS
---

1 garlic clove, peeled
2 (15-ounce) cans kidney beans, rinsed and drained
1 egg
1/3 cup shredded carrots
1/3 cup plain bread crumbs

3 scallions, white and light green parts only, thinly sliced
1 teaspoon chili powder
1/4 teaspoon salt
6 whole wheat buns
6 lettuce leaves
1/2 cup salsa

In a food processor, with the motor running, add the garlic. Add beans and egg and pulse until slightly chunky. Transfer to a bowl and stir in carrots, bread crumbs, scallions, chili powder, and salt. Form into six patties.

Coat a large skillet with nonstick cooking spray. Cook burgers for 3 to 4 minutes per side, or until cooked through and lightly crusted. Serve on whole wheat buns with lettuce and salsa.

For more nutrients, choose deeply colored lettuce leaves like red leaf or romaine. In general, the more colorful the vegetables and fruits, the more packed they are with antioxidants and phytochemicals.

Per Serving	
Calories	285
Calories from Fat	40
Total Fat	4.5 g
Saturated Fat	0.9 g
Trans Fat	0.0 g
Polyunsaturated Fat	1.1 g
Monounsaturated Fat	1.7 g
Cholesterol	35 mg
Sodium	650 mg
Total Carbohydrate	49 g
Dietary Fiber	9 g
Sugars	7 g
Protein	15 g

LAMB BURGERS WITH TOMATO–OLIVE RELISH

*For a change of pace, try a lamb burger topped with a tangy chunky relish
brimming with tomato, olives, and feta cheese.
Mint gives the burger a freshness that complements the cumin.*

SERVES 4 / PREP TIME: 15 MINUTES OR LESS / TOTAL TIME: 30 MINUTES OR LESS

1 pound ground lamb
2 tablespoons finely chopped fresh mint
1/2 teaspoon ground cumin
1/4 teaspoon salt
1/4 teaspoon coarsely ground black
  pepper
3 tablespoons nonfat plain yogurt

1 tablespoon fresh lemon juice
1 teaspoon honey
1 garlic clove, minced
1/2 cup quartered cherry tomatoes
1/4 cup chopped Kalamata olives
1/4 cup crumbled feta cheese
2 (6- to 7-inch) whole wheat pitas,
  halved

In a bowl, combine lamb, mint, cumin, salt, and pepper. Form into four patties.

Coat a large skillet with nonstick cooking spray. Over medium-high heat, cook burgers for 4 minutes per side, or until cooked through.

Meanwhile, in a bowl, combine yogurt, lemon juice, honey, and garlic. Add tomatoes, olives, and feta and stir to combine.

Place a burger in the pocket of each pita half and top with relish.

For added flavor, cook burgers
on an outdoor or indoor grill.

Per Serving	
Calories	335
Calories from Fat	170
Total Fat	19.0 g
Saturated Fat	7.6 g
Trans Fat	0.1 g
Polyunsaturated Fat	1.6 g
Monounsaturated Fat	7.6 g
Cholesterol	85 mg
Sodium	430 mg
Total Carbohydrate	20 g
Dietary Fiber	2 g
Sugars	4 g
Protein	24 g

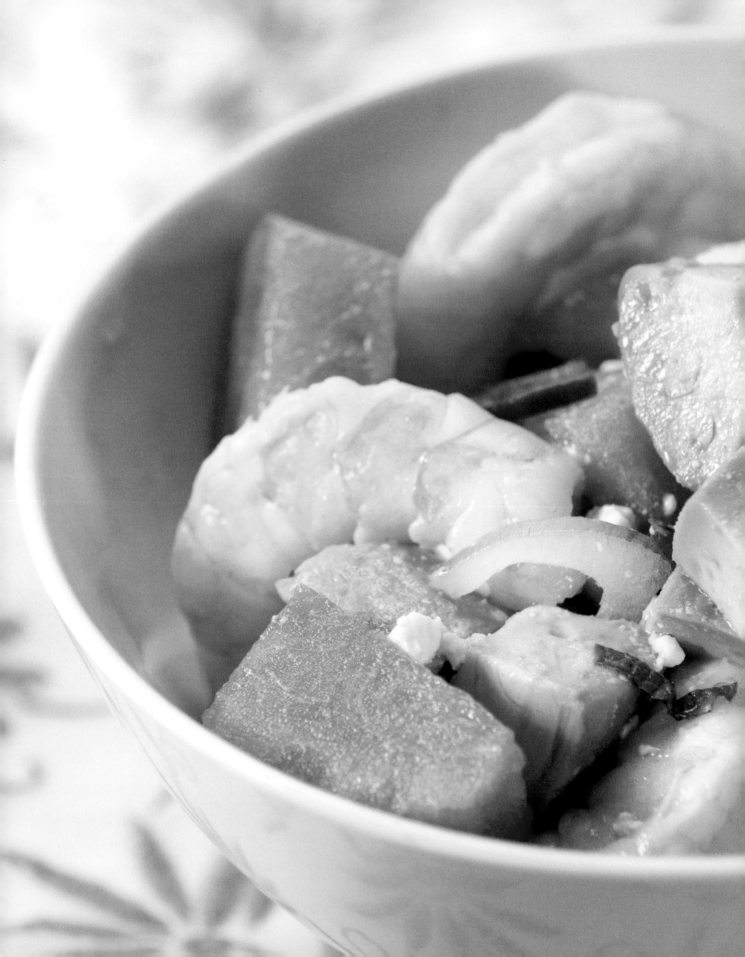

SHRIMP, WATERMELON, AND AVOCADO SALAD

Recently, watermelon has been a breakout fruit at the dinner table, being paired with all sorts of savory ingredients for unexpected tastes and textures. This refreshing salad marries the sweet and succulent melon with creamy avocado, cooked shrimp, and lots of flavorful extras, including spicy jalapeños, pungent red onion, and aromatic mint.

To prevent the salad from getting mushy, blot excess liquid from the watermelon and shrimp before combining.

For easier preparation, buy precut melon at the supermarket's produce department and precooked shrimp at the seafood counter.

SERVES 4 / PREP TIME: 15 MINUTES OR LESS / TOTAL TIME: 15 MINUTES OR LESS

---

1 pound cooked peeled and deveined shrimp

4 cups watermelon, cut into 1-inch pieces

1/4 red onion, very thinly sliced

1/4 cup thinly sliced fresh mint

1 jalapeño, halved lengthwise, seeded, and very thinly sliced

1 avocado, peeled and cut into 1/2-inch pieces

Juice of 1 lemon

1 tablespoon extra–virgin olive oil

1 teaspoon honey

1/4 teaspoon salt

1/4 teaspoon freshly ground black pepper

1/4 cup crumbled feta cheese or goat cheese

With a paper towel, blot dry shrimp and watermelon and place in a bowl. Add onion, mint, jalapeño, and avocado and stir gently to combine.

In a bowl, combine lemon juice, oil, honey, salt, and pepper. Add to salad and toss gently to combine. Top with feta cheese.

Avocados are a good source of heart-healthy monounsaturated fats. A ripe avocado will yield to gentle pressure from your hand. Store unripened avocados at room temperature in a paper bag. Once ripened, they will keep for 2 to 5 days, or longer if stored in the refrigerator.

Per Serving	
Calories	285
Calories from Fat	110
Total Fat	12.0 g
Saturated Fat	3.0 g
Trans Fat	0.1 g
Polyunsaturated Fat	1.7 g
Monounsaturated Fat	6.9 g
Cholesterol	230 mg
Sodium	510 mg
Total Carbohydrate	19 g
Dietary Fiber	4 g
Sugars	12 g
Protein	27 g

TURKEY ROLL-UP

A roll-up reminds you to fill your sandwich with lots of veggies to give it oomph! Sliced roast turkey is just the starting place. Layers of tomatoes, greens, and peppers are the yin to the turkey's yang.

SERVES 1 / PREP TIME: 15 MINUTES OR LESS / TOTAL TIME: 15 MINUTES OR LESS

1 tablespoon mustard or honey-mustard
1 (8-inch) whole wheat tortilla
2 large slices deli-cut roast turkey
 (about 1½ ounces)
3 thin slices tomato

¼ cup chopped arugula, watercress, or
 other dark, leafy green
¼ cup chopped red or yellow bell
 pepper

Spread mustard over tortilla. Layer turkey, tomato, arugula, and bell pepper on half of the tortilla. Roll up jellyroll style, beginning with the meat side. Slice into 2-inch pieces.

Per Serving
Calories 195
 Calories from Fat 40
Total Fat . . . . 4.5 g
 Saturated Fat . . . . 0.7 g
 Trans Fat . . . . 0.0 g
 Polyunsaturated Fat . . . . 1.8 g
 Monounsaturated Fat . . . . . . 1.4 g
Cholesterol . . . . 20 mg
Sodium . . . . 815 mg
Total Carbohydrate . . . . 26 g
 Dietary Fiber . . . . 5 g
 Sugars . . . . 5 g
Protein . . . . 14 g

QUINOA AND CORN SALAD WITH ROSEMARY

Quinoa (pronounced keen-wah) is an ancient seed that acts and tastes like a whole grain. It has a mild, slightly nutty taste, is a "complete" protein with all essential amino acids, and, best of all, cooks quickly. Red quinoa—a misnomer since it's actually brown— looks very pretty in this dish, but the more common white quinoa tastes just as good.

Before cooking, rinse quinoa in a sieve under cold running water until the water runs clear to remove any residue of its bitter coating, saponin.

SERVES 8 / PREP TIME: 15 MINUTES OR LESS / TOTAL TIME: 30 MINUTES OR LESS

1 cup quinoa, rinsed
3 cups water
1 (15-ounce) can no-salt-added corn, drained
¼ cup pine nuts, toasted
3 scallions, thinly sliced
1 tomato, chopped

2 tablespoons balsamic or red wine vinegar
1 tablespoon finely chopped fresh rosemary
1 tablespoon fresh lemon juice
1 tablespoon olive oil
½ teaspoon salt
¼ teaspoon ground black pepper

In a saucepan, combine quinoa and water and bring to a boil, stirring to combine. Reduce the heat, cover, and simmer for 12 to 15 minutes, or until all water is absorbed and the seeds have opened to reveal a white curled "tail." Fluff with a fork and set aside to cool.

Meanwhile, in a bowl, combine corn, pine nuts, scallions, tomato, vinegar, rosemary, lemon juice, oil, salt, and pepper. Stir in the cooled quinoa.

Quinoa provides more protein than any grain, making it very attractive for vegetarians. It is also a source of iron, magnesium, and riboflavin.

· · · · ·

Even though nuts are full of the good kind of fat, they are also full of calories. Toasting nuts before you use them in a recipe brings out their flavor so you can use less, saving on calories without sacrificing flavor. To toast pine nuts, cook in a dry skillet until golden and aromatic, shaking frequently, or bake at 350 degrees for 3 to 8 minutes, stirring occasionally. Cool before using.

Per Serving	
Calories	160
Calories from Fat	55
Total Fat	6.0 g
Saturated Fat	0.6 g
Trans Fat	0.0 g
Polyunsaturated Fat	2.4 g
Monounsaturated Fat	2.5 g
Cholesterol	0 mg
Sodium	155 mg
Total Carbohydrate	22 g
Dietary Fiber	3 g
Sugars	4 g
Protein	5 g

QUESADILLA WITH BEANS, CORN, AND GREEN CHILES

*When you need something to fill a quesadilla and have only the
cupboard to turn to for ingredients, try this version.
Make sure to pat the corn and beans dry after draining.*

*Serve with bottled salsa, Fresh Tomato Salsa,
or Spicy Tomatillo Salsa (pages 163 and 164).*

SERVES 1 / PREP TIME: 15 MINUTES OR LESS / TOTAL TIME: 15 MINUTES OR LESS

---

2 (4-inch) corn tortillas
¼ cup canned pinto beans, rinsed,
   drained, and patted dry
¼ cup shredded reduced-fat cheddar
   or "Mexican-style" shredded cheese

1 tablespoon canned no-salt-added
   corn, drained and patted dry
1 tablespoon canned diced green
   chiles, drained

On a microwave-safe plate, top one tortilla with beans. Using the back of a fork, mash the beans into a chunky paste. Top with cheese, corn, chiles, and the remaining tortilla. Microwave on HIGH for 1 minute, or until cheese melts.

Substitute black beans or other canned beans in this recipe for a slightly different flavor.

Per Serving
Calories 200
  Calories from Fat 65
Total Fat . . . . 7.0 g
  Saturated Fat . . . . 3.7 g
  Trans Fat . . . . 0.0 g
  Polyunsaturated Fat . . . . 0.6 g
  Monounsaturated Fat . . . . . . 2.0 g
Cholesterol . . . . 20 mg
Sodium . . . . 285 mg
Total Carbohydrate . . . . 23 g
  Dietary Fiber . . . . 6 g
  Sugars . . . . 2 g
Protein . . . . 12 g

SPINACH, PORTOBELLO, AND ROASTED RED PEPPER SALAD

This substantial salad provides a combination of colors, tastes, and textures to tickle the taste buds. Not a blue cheese fan? Sprinkle with feta or goat cheese crumbles.

SERVES 4 / PREP TIME: 30 MINUTES OR LESS / TOTAL TIME: 30 MINUTES OR LESS

2 tablespoons extra–virgin olive oil
2 tablespoons fresh lemon juice
1 teaspoon Dijon mustard
1 garlic clove, minced
½ teaspoon granulated sugar
½ teaspoon Italian seasoning
2 portobello mushrooms, stems removed
1 red bell pepper, seeded and halved

1 (5- or 6-ounce) bag baby spinach, tough stems removed
2 tablespoons golden raisins
2 tablespoons dried and sweetened cranberries, such as Craisins
¼ red onion, thinly sliced
¼ cup chickpeas, rinsed and drained
2 tablespoons crumbled blue cheese
1 tablespoon pine nuts, toasted

Position one oven rack 4 to 6 inches from the heat and the other in the middle of the oven and preheat the broiler. Lightly coat two foil-lined, rimmed baking sheets with nonstick cooking spray.

In a bowl, combine the oil, lemon juice, mustard, garlic, sugar, and Italian seasoning.

Brush both sides of the mushrooms with dressing and place gill side down on a baking sheet. Place the bell pepper, cut side down, on the other baking sheet. Lightly press or cut it open so it lies flat. Put the bell pepper on the top shelf and the mushrooms on the middle shelf. Cook for 3 to 4 minutes. Turn the mushrooms and cook for 3 to 5 minutes, or until mushrooms are tender and bell pepper is charred. Remove from the oven and set mushrooms aside to cool. Fold the foil over the pepper and set aside to steam as it cools. Cut mushrooms into ½-inch thick slices. Remove the skin from the bell pepper and discard. Thinly slice the pepper.

In a bowl, combine spinach, mushrooms, bell pepper, raisins, cranberries, onion, chickpeas, blue cheese, and the remaining dressing. Sprinkle with pine nuts.

> Salads are great choices for a light meal, but be sure to use just a light coating of dressing or you'll be adding a lot of calories.

Per Serving	
Calories	165
Calories from Fat	90
Total Fat	10.0 g
Saturated Fat	1.8 g
Trans Fat	0.0 g
Polyunsaturated Fat	1.7 g
Monounsaturated Fat	5.8 g
Cholesterol	5 mg
Sodium	140 mg
Total Carbohydrate	17 g
Dietary Fiber	3 g
Sugars	9 g
Protein	4 g

BEET, ORANGE, AND ARUGULA SALAD

A healthy bunch of beets is irresistible. Just wrap them in foil and pop them in the oven whenever you know you are going to be around for a little while. This assertive root vegetable can stand up to the peppery bite of arugula. Orange segments add softness while a touch of tangy cheese adds contrast.

This salad can be served as a main course, an appetizer, or a side dish. Because of its colorful ingredients, it looks especially festive when served on individual plates.

SERVES 4 / PREP TIME: 30 MINUTES OR LESS / TOTAL TIME: 1 HOUR AND 15 MINUTES OR LESS

2 large beets
2 tablespoons extra–virgin olive oil
2 tablespoons orange juice
2 teaspoons chopped shallot
½ teaspoon Dijon mustard
½ teaspoon granulated sugar

Pinch salt
6 cups arugula
1 to 2 oranges, peeled and segmented
4 tablespoons crumbled goat cheese or feta cheese
4 teaspoons chopped walnuts, toasted

Preheat the oven to 400 degrees.

Wrap beets well in foil and bake for 45 to 60 minutes, or until a knife can easily pierce them. Set aside to cool. Peel off outside layer and cut into wedges on a paper towel lined plate.

Meanwhile, combine oil, orange juice, shallot, mustard, sugar, and salt and stir well to combine.

In a bowl, combine arugula with 2 tablespoons of the dressing. Divide on individual plates. Arrange beet wedges and orange sections in a fan. Sprinkle with goat cheese and walnuts. Drizzle with the remaining dressing if desired.

Each beet provides 20 percent of the Recommended Dietary Allowance of folate, as well as providing iron.

Per Serving	
Calories	115
Calories from Fat	65
Total Fat	7.0 g
Saturated Fat	2.0 g
Trans Fat	0.1 g
Polyunsaturated Fat	1.7 g
Monounsaturated Fat	3.2 g
Cholesterol	10 mg
Sodium	155 mg
Total Carbohydrate	11 g
Dietary Fiber	2 g
Sugars	7 g
Protein	4 g

ROAST BEEF ROLL-UP

A rolled sandwich packed with extra vegetables is a great way to satisfy a red meat craving without overdoing it. Horseradish stands up to roast beef without overwhelming it. Make your own spicy mayo dip or, for a different spin, use a packaged wasabi mayo blend or try the recipe from Wasabi Salmon Burgers on page 5.

SERVES 1 / PREP TIME: 15 MINUTES OR LESS / TOTAL TIME: 15 MINUTES OR LESS

1 tablespoon good-quality light
    mayonnaise, such as Hellmann's
1 teaspoon prepared horseradish
1 (8-inch) whole wheat tortilla

2 large slices deli-cut roast beef (about
    1½ ounces)
5 very thin slices peeled cucumber
10 to 15 fresh spinach leaves
¼ cup shredded carrots

In a bowl, combine mayonnaise and horseradish. Spread over tortilla. Layer roast beef, cucumber, spinach, and carrots on half of the tortilla. Roll up jellyroll style, beginning with the meat side. Slice into 2-inch pieces.

Per Serving
Calories 250
    Calories from Fat 80
Total Fat . . . . 9.0 g
    Saturated Fat . . . . 1.7 g
    Trans Fat . . . . 0.0 g
    Polyunsaturated Fat . . . . 3.6 g
    Monounsaturated Fat . . . . . . 2.9 g
Cholesterol . . . . 30 mg
Sodium . . . . 635 mg
Total Carbohydrate . . . . 25 g
    Dietary Fiber . . . . 4 g
    Sugars . . . . 4 g
Protein . . . . 15 g

WHEAT BERRY SALAD WITH ALMONDS AND DRIED CHERRIES

Nutty, wholesome wheat berries—the whole wheat kernel, minus the inedible outer hull—taste delicious year-round, but seem especially hearty on winter days.

While wheat berries, sold in bulk in health food stores, might not be that familiar, once you try them you may find them surprisingly addictive. This salad, with nuts, cucumber, and dried cherries, is just one combination. You can substitute apples or oranges for the cherries and celery or fennel for the cucumbers.

Before cooking, rinse the wheat berries under cold water. Cooking time can vary depending on the variety, so begin checking for doneness after 1 hour. They should still have some chew to them after cooking.

SERVES 6 / PREP TIME: 15 MINUTES OR LESS / TOTAL TIME: 2 HOURS OR LESS

---

1 cup dried wheat berries, rinsed

3 cups water

2 scallions, thinly sliced

1/2 cucumber, peeled, seeded, and chopped

1/3 cup dried cherries

2 tablespoons cider vinegar

1 1/2 tablespoons olive oil

1 tablespoon chopped fresh Italian parsley

1/4 teaspoon salt

1/4 teaspoon ground black pepper

1/3 cup sliced almonds, toasted

In a medium saucepan, combine wheat berries and water and bring to a boil, stirring to combine. Reduce the heat, cover, and simmer for 1 to 1 1/2 hours, or until wheat berries are tender and all or most of the liquid is absorbed. Remove from heat, drain if necessary, and cool to room temperature.

Meanwhile, in a bowl, combine scallions, cucumber, cherries, vinegar, oil, parsley, salt, and pepper. Stir in the cooled wheat berries and almonds.

Per Serving	
Calories	200
Calories from Fat	70
Total Fat	8.0 g
Saturated Fat	0.9 g
Trans Fat	0.0 g
Polyunsaturated Fat	1.5 g
Monounsaturated Fat	5.1 g
Cholesterol	0 mg
Sodium	100 mg
Total Carbohydrate	29 g
Dietary Fiber	5 g
Sugars	5 g
Protein	7 g

Wheat berries are whole grains high in protein and fiber.

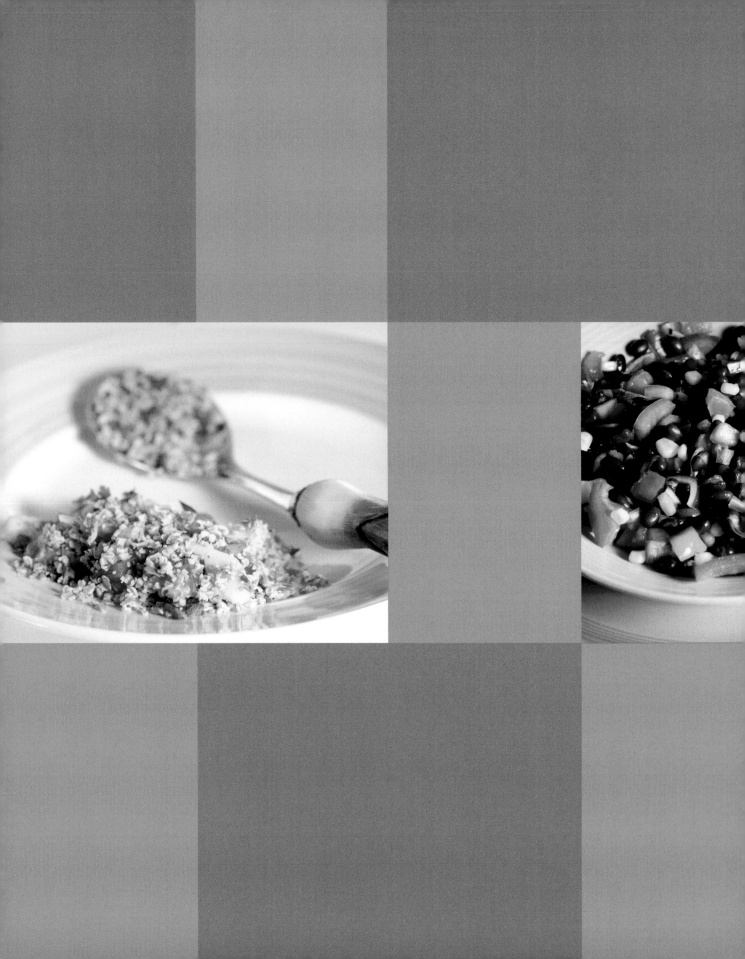

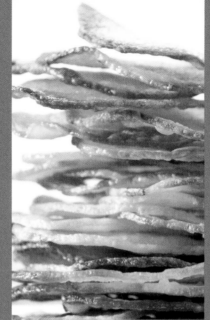

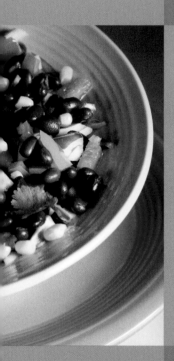

SIDES

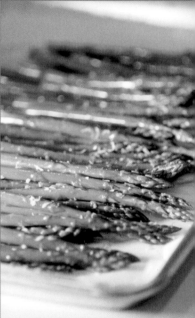

These side dishes will take center stage as they round out your meal and make it that much more enjoyable. Dazzle your palate with something new and different, or relax with your classic comfort food favorites. Adding a rainbow of colors and an extravaganza of tastes and textures, these dishes deliver!

CHUNKY VEGETABLE SALAD

In the warmer months, when produce is in its prime,
try a salad that celebrates the integrity of each vegetable.
This colorful cut-up veggie mix, with large chunks of crunchy cucumber,
bell peppers, and fennel, is a welcome change from traditional leafy greens.

A splash of white balsamic vinaigrette and a
smattering of dill is all you need to dress it.

SERVES 10 / PREP TIME: 15 MINUTES OR LESS / TOTAL TIME: 15 MINUTES OR LESS

---

3 ripe tomatoes, seeded and cut into
  1-inch pieces
1 large cucumber, peeled, seeded, and
  cut into 1-inch pieces
1 red bell pepper, seeded and cut into
  1-inch pieces
1 yellow bell pepper, seeded and cut
  into 1-inch pieces

1 fennel bulb, cored and cut into
  1-inch pieces
1 tablespoon finely chopped fresh dill
1 tablespoon white balsamic vinegar
1 tablespoon extra–virgin olive oil
Pinch granulated sugar
Salt and freshly ground black pepper

In a bowl, combine tomatoes, cucumber, both bell peppers, fennel, and dill.
  In a bowl, combine vinegar, oil, and sugar. Season with salt and pepper.
  Drizzle over salad and toss to combine.

White balsamic vinegar has a slightly milder flavor
than red. It is found in the vinegar section of most
supermarkets. Substitute regular balsamic vinegar
for white if you have trouble finding it.

Per Serving	
Calories	40
Calories from Fat	15
Total Fat	1.5 g
Saturated Fat	0.2 g
Trans Fat	0.0 g
Polyunsaturated Fat	0.2 g
Monounsaturated Fat	1.0 g
Cholesterol	0 mg
Sodium	15 mg
Total Carbohydrate	6 g
Dietary Fiber	2 g
Sugars	3 g
Protein	1 g

CARROT–RAISIN–APPLE SALAD

The surprising sweetness of apple and crunch of roasted sesame seeds give unexpected dimension to this traditional slaw. Instead of wallowing in mayonnaise, this version uses only enough to lightly coat the ingredients and hold the salad together. Use bagged matchstick-cut carrots for easier prep.

You can make this ahead, but wait until just before serving to add the sunflower seeds.

SERVES 6 / PREP TIME: 15 MINUTES OR LESS / TOTAL TIME: 15 MINUTES OR LESS

2 cups matchstick-cut or shredded carrots
¼ cup raisins
1 Granny Smith apple, chopped

2 tablespoons good-quality light mayonnaise, such as Hellmann's
1 tablespoon fresh lemon juice
2 tablespoons roasted sunflower seed kernels

In a bowl, combine carrots, raisins, apple, mayonnaise, and lemon juice. Sprinkle with sunflower seeds.

Carrots are a vitamin A powerhouse!
. . . . .
Raisins provide fiber, potassium, iron, and antioxidants.

Per Serving
Calories 95
    Calories from Fat 25
Total Fat . . . . 3.0 g
    Saturated Fat . . . . 0.4 g
    Trans Fat . . . . 0.0 g
    Polyunsaturated Fat . . . . 1.8 g
    Monounsaturated Fat . . . . . . 0.6 g
Cholesterol . . . . 0 mg
Sodium . . . . 70 mg
Total Carbohydrate . . . . 18 g
    Dietary Fiber . . . . 3 g
    Sugars . . . . 12 g
Protein . . . . 1 g

OVEN-BAKED POTATO CHIPS

Homemade potato chips are the ultimate crowd pleaser. Made with just a bit of olive oil, they can be enjoyed without the fat and guilt of packaged chips.

Because the potatoes need to be sliced very thinly for even baking, a mandoline (a handheld slicer) or a very sharp knife is recommended. Inexpensive mandolines can be bought at kitchen stores and some supermarkets. Oddly, even when uniformly sliced, the chips still cook at slightly different rates, so watch carefully and remove chips as they are done, leaving the others to continue cooking.

Line your baking sheets with parchment paper to speed cleanup and prevent sticking.

SERVES 4 / PREP TIME: 15 MINUTES OR LESS / TOTAL TIME: 45 MINUTES OR LESS

---

1 tablespoon olive oil
2 large potatoes, peeled and sliced ⅛-inch thick
Kosher or sea salt

Preheat the oven to 400 degrees. Lightly brush two rimmed baking sheets with oil and sprinkle with salt. Place potato slices in a single layer on the baking sheets. Brush tops of potatoes with oil and sprinkle with salt.

Bake for 15 to 25 minutes, or until golden, checking often after 10 minutes and removing chips that have browned. Transfer to a plate lined with paper towels.

For a special treat, brush potato slices with rosemary oil from the recipe for Rosemary Popcorn (page 153).

Per Serving	
Calories	105
Calories from Fat	30
Total Fat	3.5 g
Saturated Fat	0.5 g
Trans Fat	0.0 g
Polyunsaturated Fat	0.4 g
Monounsaturated Fat	2.5 g
Cholesterol	0 mg
Sodium	0 mg
Total Carbohydrate	18 g
Dietary Fiber	2 g
Sugars	1 g
Protein	1 g

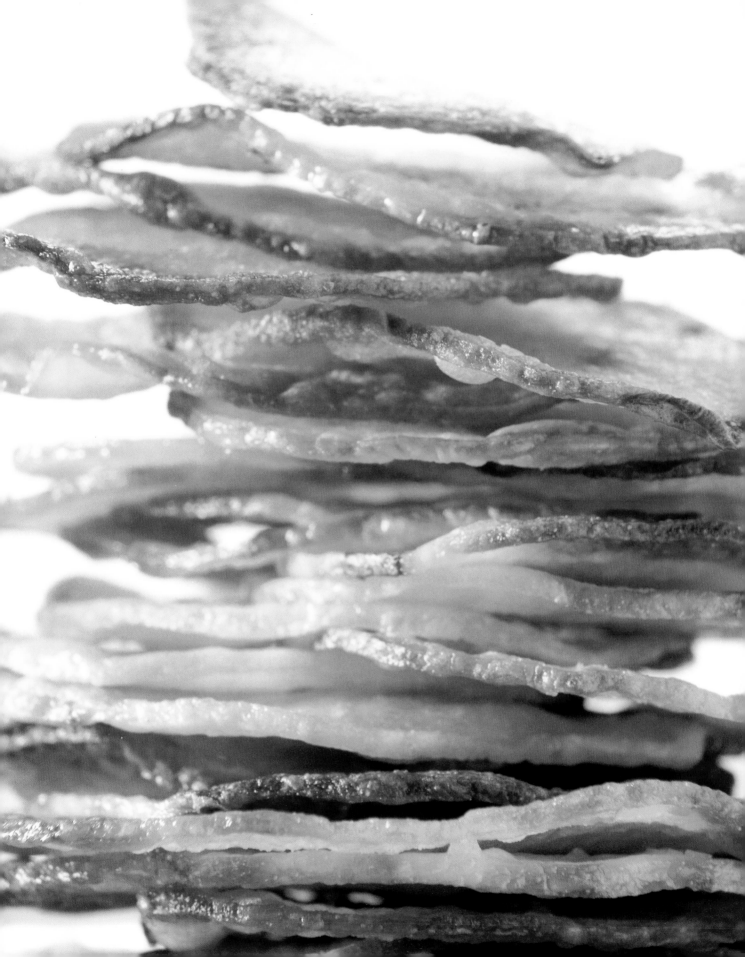

SWEET POTATO FRIES

Sweet potato fries are an ideal side dish or snack.
If you're in the mood for something savory, sprinkle them with a Cajun
seasoning blend. For something sweet, use a cinnamon-sugar mix.

Line your baking sheet with aluminum foil or parchment paper
to speed cleanup and prevent sticking.

SERVES 2 / PREP TIME: 15 MINUTES OR LESS / TOTAL TIME: 30 MINUTES OR LESS

---

1 sweet potato   Kosher or sea salt
2 teaspoons olive oil

Preheat the oven to 425 degrees. Lightly coat a rimmed baking sheet with nonstick cooking spray.

Cut potatoes in half lengthwise and then in wedges. Brush wedges with oil and sprinkle with salt. Place on the baking sheet.

Bake for 10 minutes, turn wedges over, and bake for 5 to 10 minutes, or until easily pierced by a knife and golden.

Sweet potatoes are filled with beta-carotene
and are a good source of fiber.
. . . . .
Most chefs prefer the cleaner taste of kosher and
sea salt. In fact, it's all most professional chefs use.

Per Serving	
Calories	105
Calories from Fat	40
Total Fat	4.5 g
Saturated Fat	0.6 g
Trans Fat	0.0 g
Polyunsaturated Fat	0.5 g
Monounsaturated Fat	3.3 g
Cholesterol	0 mg
Sodium	25 mg
Total Carbohydrate	15 g
Dietary Fiber	2 g
Sugars	5 g
Protein	1 g

CARAWAY COLE SLAW

This slaw is equally good as a side salad or as a topping to a sandwich. Unlike other types of slaw, it has just enough dressing to coat the cabbage, but it isn't swimming in excess. Caraway seeds add a distinctive note.

SERVES 4 / PREP TIME: 15 MINUTES OR LESS
TOTAL TIME: 1 HOUR AND 15 MINUTES INCLUDING REFRIGERATION TIME

2 tablespoons good-quality light mayonnaise, such as Hellmann's

2 tablespoons nonfat plain yogurt

2 teaspoons granulated sugar

1 tablespoon white vinegar

4 cups shredded cabbage or cole slaw mix

1 teaspoon caraway seeds

Salt and freshly ground black pepper

In a bowl, combine mayonnaise, yogurt, sugar, and vinegar. Add cabbage and caraway seeds and toss to combine. Season with salt and pepper. Refrigerate for 1 hour or more.

If you have leftover cabbage mix, make Moo Shu Chicken Lettuce Wraps (page 55).

Per Serving

Calories	55
Calories from Fat	20
Total Fat	2.5 g
Saturated Fat	0.4 g
Trans Fat	0.0 g
Polyunsaturated Fat	1.3 g
Monounsaturated Fat	0.6 g
Cholesterol	5 mg
Sodium	80 mg
Total Carbohydrate	7 g
Dietary Fiber	2 g
Sugars	5 g
Protein	1 g

GARLIC MASHED POTATOES

Mashed potatoes don't have to be enriched with heavy cream and gobs of butter to taste good. Here, buttermilk is the surprise ingredient, keeping these potatoes both good-tasting and good for you.

Because Yukon Gold and red potatoes have thin skins, you don't need to peel them before cooking. This fortifies the dish with extra nutrients found in potato skins.

SERVES 4 / PREP TIME: 15 MINUTES OR LESS / TOTAL TIME: 30 MINUTES OR LESS

¾ pound small Yukon Gold or red potatoes, cut into 2-inch pieces
3 garlic cloves
½ cup nonfat or reduced-fat buttermilk, heated

1 tablespoon butter, cut into pieces
Salt and freshly ground black pepper

In a saucepan, cover potatoes with 1 inch of water and bring to a boil. Reduce the heat and simmer for 10 minutes, stirring occasionally. Add garlic and simmer for 5 to 10 minutes, or until potatoes are tender and a knife can easily pierce them.

Drain potatoes and garlic and return to the pot. Add buttermilk and butter and beat with an electric mixer until smooth. Season generously with salt and pepper.

Potatoes are a good source of potassium.
. . . . .
Buttermilk adds a tangy flavor and richness, even though it is low in fat.

Per Serving	
Calories	110
Calories from Fat	25
Total Fat	3.0 g
Saturated Fat	2.0 g
Trans Fat	0.0 g
Polyunsaturated Fat	0.2 g
Monounsaturated Fat	0.8 g
Cholesterol	10 mg
Sodium	55 mg
Total Carbohydrate	19 g
Dietary Fiber	2 g
Sugars	3 g
Protein	3 g

ARUGULA AND PARMIGIANO–REGGIANO SALAD

This salad can be stunning, but a simple salad such as this one is only as good as its ingredients. The key is in choosing super-fresh greens, extra–virgin olive oil, and Parmigiano–Reggiano or other high-quality block Parmesan cheese.

Arugula, a peppery-tasting leafy green, needs only a light coating of olive oil and a squirt of lemon. A topping of shaved Parmigiano–Reggiano cheese adds saltiness and pungency.

To transform this salad into a main course, top the greens with sliced grilled chicken or steak.

SERVES 4 / PREP TIME: 15 MINUTES OR LESS / TOTAL TIME: 15 MINUTES OR LESS

6 cups arugula
1 tablespoon extra–virgin olive oil
1 to 2 tablespoons lemon juice, or to taste

Kosher or sea salt and freshly ground black pepper
1 ounce Parmigiano–Reggiano cheese, shaved into 1-inch pieces

In a bowl, combine arugula and oil. Add lemon juice and season generously with salt and pepper. Top with shaved cheese.

A vegetable peeler delivers paper-thin slices of cheese.

. . . . .

For a more colorful salad, add strips of roasted red pepper. You can buy them already roasted, or roast your own: see page 95 for instructions to make them yourself.

Per Serving
Calories 65
  Calories from Fat 45
Total Fat . . . . 5.0 g
  Saturated Fat . . . . 1.6 g
  Trans Fat . . . . 0.0 g
  Polyunsaturated Fat . . . . . . 0.5 g
  Monounsaturated Fat . . . . . . 3.0 g
Cholesterol . . . . 5 mg
Sodium . . . . 65 mg
Total Carbohydrate . . . . 1 g
  Dietary Fiber . . . . 0 g
  Sugars . . . . 1 g
Protein . . . . 3 g

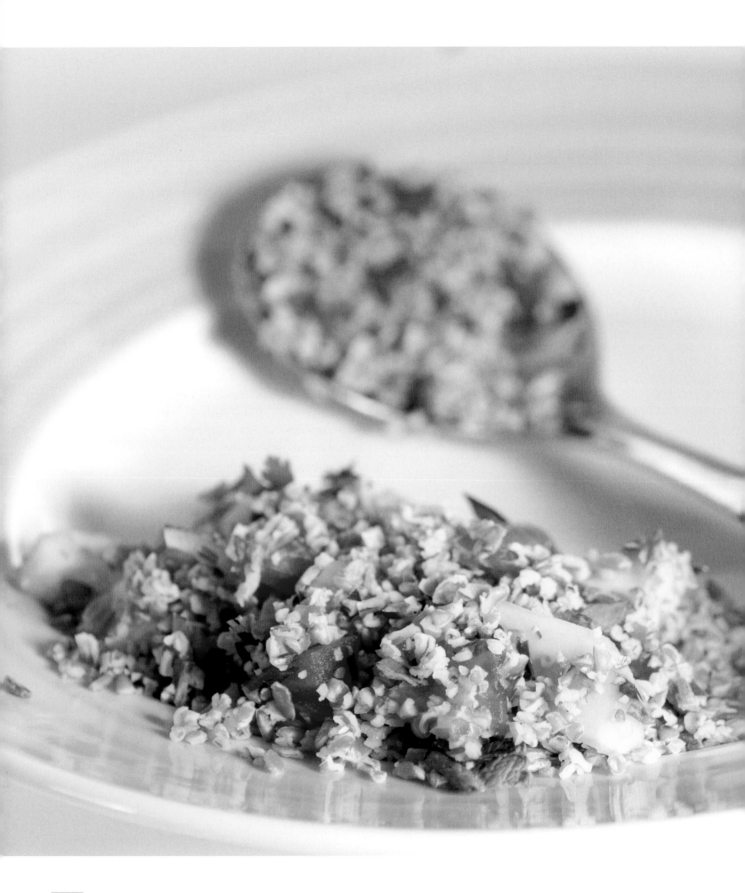

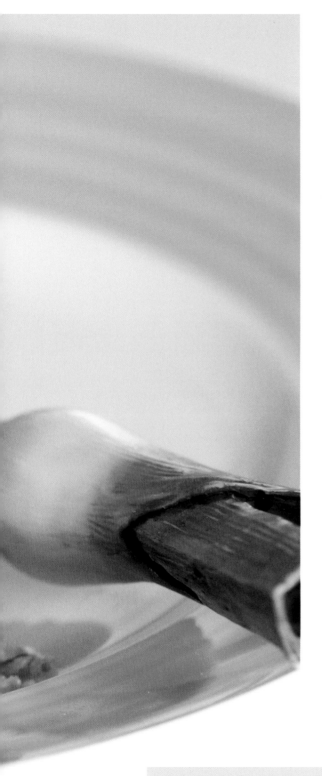

TABBOULEH SALAD

This traditional Middle Eastern salad is full of fresh veggies and bulgur. Unlike some other grains, bulgur needs only to be "rehydrated" with boiling water and is ready in about 30 minutes. In contrast to some other versions of tabbouleh, this recipe is light on oil.

Because this recipe feeds a crowd, it is a great dish to bring to a potluck.

SERVES 10 / PREP TIME: 30 MINUTES OR LESS / TOTAL TIME: 1 HOUR AND 30 MINUTES INCLUDING REFRIGERATION TIME

1$\frac{1}{2}$ cups bulgur
1$\frac{1}{2}$ cups boiling water
3 plum tomatoes, seeded and chopped
1 cucumber, peeled, seeded, and chopped
1 cup chopped fresh Italian parsley
$\frac{1}{2}$ cup finely chopped red onion
2 tablespoons chopped fresh mint
2 tablespoons extra-virgin olive oil
$\frac{1}{3}$ cup fresh lemon juice, or to taste
Salt and freshly ground black pepper

In a heatproof bowl, combine bulgur and water for 30 minutes (if mixture absorbs the water too quickly, add more water 1 tablespoon at a time). Add tomatoes, cucumber, parsley, onion, mint, oil, and lemon juice. Season with salt and pepper. Refrigerate for 1 hour or more.

Bulgur, also known as cracked wheat, is one of the most fiber-rich grains.

Per Serving	
Calories	110
Calories from Fat	25
Total Fat	3.0 g
Saturated Fat	0.4 g
Trans Fat	0.0 g
Polyunsaturated Fat	0.4 g
Monounsaturated Fat	2.1 g
Cholesterol	0 mg
Sodium	10 mg
Total Carbohydrate	19 g
Dietary Fiber	5 g
Sugars	1 g
Protein	3 g

GREENS AND HERB SALAD

It's amazing how something as simple as the addition of fresh herbs can add intensity to a side salad. Mark this recipe for the warmer months when herbs are growing abundantly.

SERVES 4 / PREP TIME: 15 MINUTES OR LESS / TOTAL TIME: 15 MINUTES OR LESS

1 tablespoon minced shallot
1 tablespoon extra–virgin olive oil
2 teaspoons red wine vinegar
6 cups mixed baby greens
1/2 cup chopped fresh herbs, such as parsley, cilantro, mint, basil, dill, and/or chervil

1/2 cucumber, peeled, seeded, and chopped
Kosher or sea salt and freshly ground black pepper

In a bowl, combine shallot, oil, and vinegar.

In a bowl, combine lettuce, herbs, and cucumber. Add enough dressing to lightly coat. Season with salt and pepper.

Fresh herbs, like parsley, basil, and cilantro, add brightness to salads, soups, salsas, and sauces. Store herbs in the refrigerator and use promptly.

Per Serving
Calories 45
  Calories from Fat 30
Total Fat . . . . 3.5 g
  Saturated Fat . . . . 0.5 g
  Trans Fat . . . . 0.0 g
  Polyunsaturated Fat . . . . 0.4 g
  Monounsaturated Fat . . . . . . 2.5 g
Cholesterol . . . . 0 mg
Sodium . . . . 15 mg
Total Carbohydrate . . . . 4 g
  Dietary Fiber . . . . 1 g
  Sugars . . . . 2 g
Protein . . . . 1 g

WHIPPED CIDER SWEET POTATOES

At Thanksgiving and other special occasions, it's nice to have spiffed-up sweet potatoes that aren't too cloying or heavy. Simmering sweet potatoes with apple cider imparts holiday flavors and aromas without taking a toll on your waistline.

For kids who like things a little sweeter, sprinkle with brown sugar before serving. This recipe can easily be increased for larger groups.

SERVES 4 / PREP TIME: 15 MINUTES OR LESS / TOTAL TIME: 30 MINUTES OR LESS

2 sweet potatoes (about 1¼ pounds), peeled and cut into 1-inch pieces
1½ cups apple cider

1 cinnamon stick
1 tablespoon butter, optional
Salt and freshly ground black pepper

In a saucepan, combine potatoes, cider, and cinnamon stick and bring to a boil, stirring occasionally. The liquid will not cover the potatoes entirely. Reduce the heat, partially cover, and simmer for 20 minutes, or until tender and a knife can easily pierce them, stirring occasionally. Remove cinnamon stick. Add butter and beat with an electric mixer until smooth. Season generously with salt and pepper.

Per Serving
Calories 175
  Calories from Fat 0
Total Fat . . . . 0.0 g
  Saturated Fat . . . . 0.1 g
  Trans Fat . . . . 0.0 g
  Polyunsaturated Fat . . . . 0.2 g
  Monounsaturated Fat . . . . . . 0.0 g
Cholesterol . . . . 0 mg
Sodium . . . . 20 mg
Total Carbohydrate . . . . 41 g
  Dietary Fiber . . . . 2 g
  Sugars . . . . 17 g
Protein . . . . 2 g

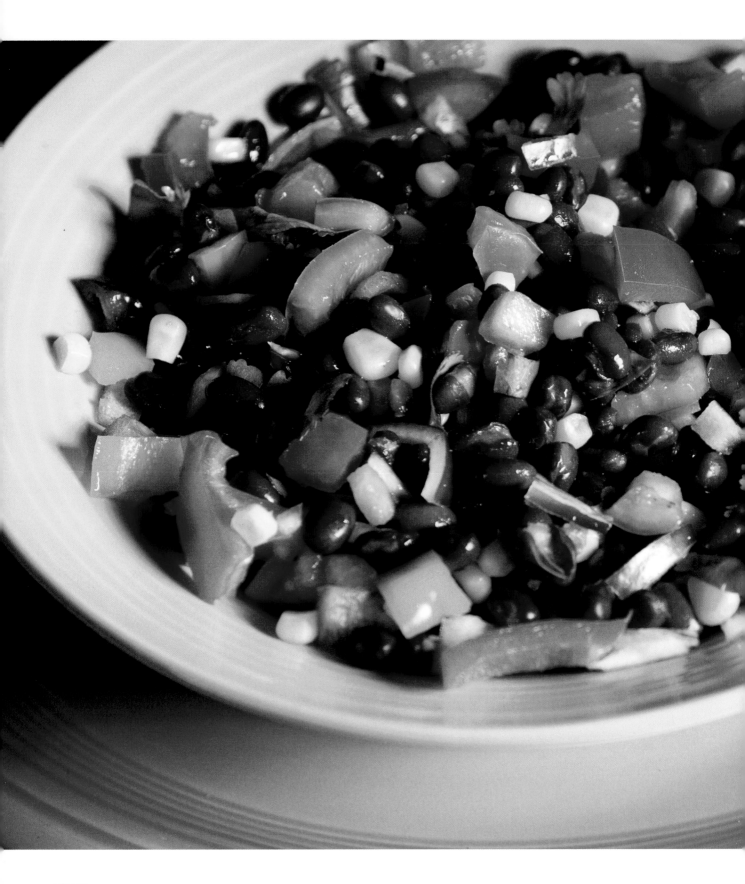

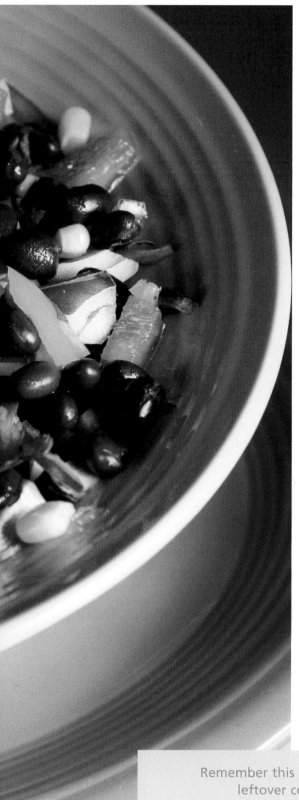

BLACK BEAN AND CORN SALAD

This salad is a great side dish for Mexican entrées or can be used as a dip for tortilla chips to start the meal. Use the measurements as a guide, but feel free to tinker.

SERVES 8 TO 10 / PREP TIME: 15 MINUTES OR LESS
TOTAL TIME: 15 MINUTES OR LESS

2 (15-ounce) cans black beans, rinsed and drained
1 cup fresh, frozen, or canned no-salt-added corn, drained
1 tomato, chopped
1 red, yellow, or green bell pepper, seeded and chopped
¹/₂ small red onion, chopped
1 jalapeño, seeded and finely chopped
2 tablespoons fresh lime juice
1 tablespoon olive oil
1 teaspoon ground cumin
Salt and freshly ground black pepper
¹/₄ cup chopped fresh cilantro

In a bowl, combine black beans, corn, tomato, bell pepper, onion, and jalapeño. In a bowl, combine lime juice, oil, and cumin and drizzle over bean mixture. Season with salt and pepper and sprinkle with cilantro.

Remember this salad when you have leftover corn on the cob.

Per Serving (for 8 servings)	
Calories	125
Calories from Fat	20
Total Fat	2.5 g
Saturated Fat	0.4 g
Trans Fat	0.0 g
Polyunsaturated Fat	0.5 g
Monounsaturated Fat	1.4 g
Cholesterol	0 mg
Sodium	80 mg
Total Carbohydrate	20 g
Dietary Fiber	7 g
Sugars	5 g
Protein	6 g

BRAISED RED CABBAGE AND APPLES

*Red cabbage is always a colorful addition to any meal,
as well as being a good source of antioxidants and vitamins A and C.*

SERVES 8 TO 10 / PREP TIME: 15 MINUTES OR LESS / TOTAL TIME: 45 MINUTES OR LESS

2 teaspoons canola oil
1 head red cabbage, quartered, cored,
  and thinly sliced
3 Granny Smith apples, peeled, cored,
  and chopped

½ cup orange juice or water
2 tablespoons cider vinegar
2 tablespoons light brown sugar,
  or to taste
Salt

In a large skillet or stockpot over medium heat, add oil. Sauté the cabbage and apples for 3 to 5 minutes. Add juice, vinegar, and sugar and sauté until cabbage begins to wilt. Cover and cook for 20 to 30 minutes, or until the cabbage is tender and the apples are soft, stirring occasionally. Season with salt.

Cruciferous vegetables—a group that includes cabbage, broccoli, cauliflower, Brussels sprouts, and kale—have compounds thought to reduce the risk of colon cancer. Include these, along with other vegetables, on your weekly shopping list.

Per Serving (for 8 servings)
Calories 85
  Calories from Fat 15
Total Fat . . . . 1.5 g
  Saturated Fat . . . . 0.1 g
  Trans Fat . . . . 0.0 g
  Polyunsaturated Fat . . . . . . 0.5 g
  Monounsaturated Fat . . . . . . 0.7 g
Cholesterol . . . . 0 mg
Sodium . . . . 15 mg
Total Carbohydrate . . . . 18 g
  Dietary Fiber . . . . 3 g
  Sugars . . . . 15 g
Protein . . . . 2 g

SAUTÉED GREEN BEANS AND GRAPE TOMATOES

Instead of serving plain steamed green beans, this side dish pairs sautéed beans with aromatic onion and garlic. A sprinkling of halved grape tomatoes completes the dish.

SERVES 4 / PREP TIME: 15 MINUTES OR LESS / TOTAL TIME: 30 MINUTES OR LESS

1 tablespoon olive oil
1 onion, halved and thinly sliced
4 garlic cloves, thinly sliced
¾ pound green beans, trimmed

¼ cup water
½ cup halved grape tomatoes
Salt and freshly ground black pepper

In a large skillet over medium heat, add oil. Sauté the onion for 7 to 10 minutes, or until softened and beginning to turn golden. Add garlic and sauté for 1 minute. Add green beans and water, cover, and cook for 5 to 7 minutes or until crisp-tender, stirring occasionally. Add tomatoes and sauté for 1 minute. Season with salt and pepper.

Per Serving	
Calories	80
Calories from Fat	30
Total Fat	3.5 g
Saturated Fat	0.5 g
Trans Fat	0.0 g
Polyunsaturated Fat	0.5 g
Monounsaturated Fat	2.5 g
Cholesterol	0 mg
Sodium	0 mg
Total Carbohydrate	11 g
Dietary Fiber	3 g
Sugars	3 g
Protein	2 g

BROWN RICE PILAF

Brown rice doesn't have to be boring. Add some aromatic spices and dried fruit for a side dish that will brighten up a simple roast or chicken breast.

Since cooking directions for each brand of rice can vary slightly, follow the package directions for the amount of liquid needed for 1 cup of rice.

SERVES 6 / PREP TIME: 15 MINUTES OR LESS / TOTAL TIME: 45 MINUTES OR LESS

---

1 tablespoon olive oil
1 small onion, finely chopped
1 cup brown rice
¼ teaspoon ground ginger
¼ teaspoon ground cinnamon

2¼ cups reduced–sodium chicken broth
⅓ cup chopped dried apricots
⅓ cup currants, raisins, or golden raisins
⅓ cup dried and sweetened cranberries, such as Craisins

In a saucepot over medium-high heat, add oil. Sauté the onion for 5 to 8 minutes, or until softened. Add rice, ginger, and cinnamon and sauté for 1 minute.

Add broth and bring to a boil, stirring to combine. Reduce the heat to low, cover, and cook for 30 minutes (or according to package directions), or until the broth is absorbed and the rice is tender. Stir in the apricots, currants, and cranberries. Cover and let sit for 1 minute.

Per Serving	
Calories	220
Calories from Fat	30
Total Fat	3.5 g
Saturated Fat	0.5 g
Trans Fat	0.0 g
Polyunsaturated Fat	0.6 g
Monounsaturated Fat	2.0 g
Cholesterol	0 mg
Sodium	195 mg
Total Carbohydrate	44 g
Dietary Fiber	4 g
Sugars	17 g
Protein	4 g

BASMATI RICE AND CHICKPEA PILAF

Add fiber and nutrients to basmati rice by adding dried fruit and legumes. To add extra flavor, add 1 teaspoon ground cumin or ½ teaspoon ground cinnamon.

SERVES 4 / PREP TIME: 15 MINUTES OR LESS / TOTAL TIME: 45 MINUTES OR LESS

2 teaspoons olive oil
½ cup chopped onion
1 cup basmati rice

2 cups reduced–sodium chicken broth
¾ cup currants or raisins
¾ cup chickpeas, rinsed and drained

In a saucepan over medium heat, add oil. Sauté the onion for 5 to 8 minutes, or until softened. Add rice and sauté for 1 minute.

Add broth and bring to a boil, stirring to combine. Reduce the heat to low, cover, and cook for 20 to 30 minutes (or according to package directions), or until the broth is absorbed and the rice is tender. Stir in currants and chickpeas. Cover and let sit 1 minute.

The Hindi word "basmati" means fragrant, and refers to the nut-like flavor and aroma of this long grain rice. Cultivated in India and Pakistan for thousands of years, the grains of basmati rice stay firm and separate after cooking instead of getting sticky.

Per Serving	
Calories	330
Calories from Fat	30
Total Fat	3.5 g
Saturated Fat	0.5 g
Trans Fat	0.0 g
Polyunsaturated Fat	0.7 g
Monounsaturated Fat	2.0 g
Cholesterol	0 mg
Sodium	310 mg
Total Carbohydrate	66 g
Dietary Fiber	4 g
Sugars	25 g
Protein	8 g

LEMON-ROASTED ASPARAGUS

Roasted asparagus is a welcome addition to any meal. Choose uniform stalks of medium thickness for even cooking. Adjust time depending on the size of the asparagus.

Line your baking sheet with aluminum foil or parchment paper to speed cleanup.

SERVES 4 / PREP TIME: 15 MINUTES OR LESS / TOTAL TIME: 15 MINUTES OR LESS

---

1 lemon

1 pound asparagus, tough ends removed

1 tablespoon olive oil

Salt and freshly ground black pepper

Preheat the oven to 450 degrees.

Grate the zest and squeeze the juice from the lemon.

On a rimmed baking sheet, place asparagus in a single layer. Drizzle with oil and roll asparagus to lightly coat. Sprinkle with lemon zest, salt, and pepper.

Roast for 5 to 7 minutes, remove from the oven, and roll asparagus for even cooking. Roast for 2 to 4 minutes, or until just tender. Drizzle with 1 teaspoon lemon juice.

Asparagus is filled with folate, iron, and many antioxidants.

Per Serving	
Calories	50
Calories from Fat	30
Total Fat	3.5 g
Saturated Fat	0.5 g
Trans Fat	0.0 g
Polyunsaturated Fat	0.4 g
Monounsaturated Fat	2.5 g
Cholesterol	0 mg
Sodium	10 mg
Total Carbohydrate	4 g
Dietary Fiber	1 g
Sugars	1 g
Protein	2 g

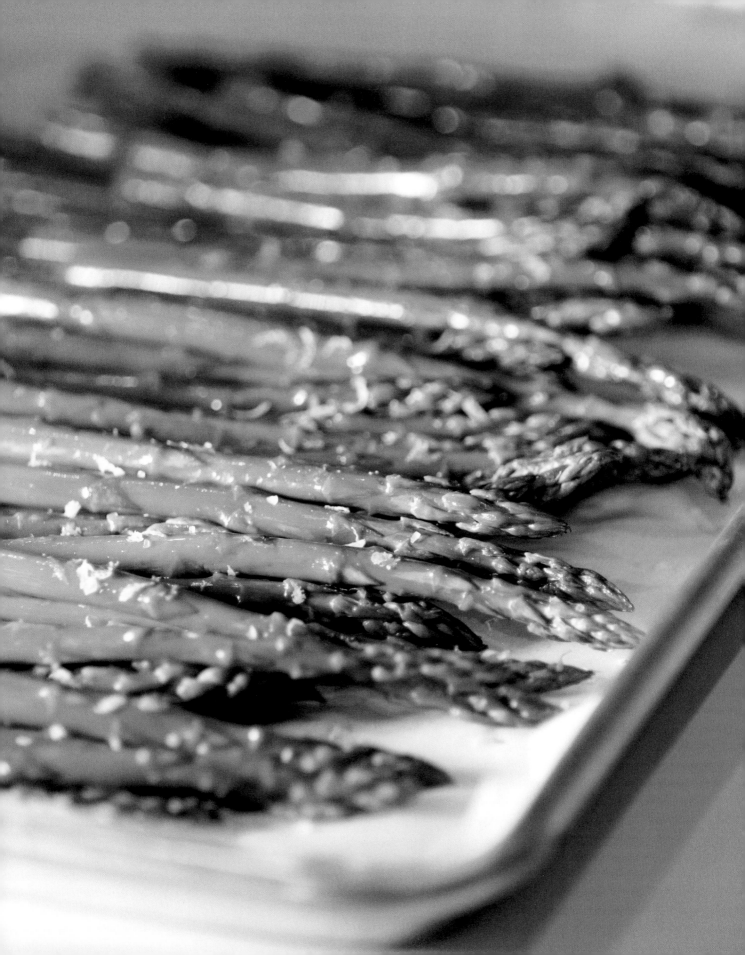

ORANGE–GLAZED BABY CARROTS

Orange marmalade adds a surprising hint of citrus and sweetness to glazed carrots. Bagged baby carrots are a great no-prep veggie.

SERVES 4 / PREP TIME: 15 MINUTES OR LESS / TOTAL TIME: 30 MINUTES OR LESS

1 (1-pound) bag baby carrots
1 cup water
2 tablespoons orange marmalade

1 tablespoon butter
½ teaspoon salt

In a 10-inch skillet over medium-high heat, combine carrots, water, marmalade, butter, and salt. Cook for 20 to 30 minutes, stirring occasionally, until all of the water has evaporated and the carrots are glazed and tender.

Per Serving	
Calories	95
Calories from Fat	25
Total Fat	3.0 g
Saturated Fat	1.8 g
Trans Fat	0.0 g
Polyunsaturated Fat	0.2 g
Monounsaturated Fat	0.8 g
Cholesterol	10 mg
Sodium	385 mg
Total Carbohydrate	18 g
Dietary Fiber	4 g
Sugars	10 g
Protein	1 g

EGGPLANT SPREAD

*This veggie spread is a great side dish for fish or Greek entrées.
It can also be served with Cheesy Pita Crisps (page 152) as an appetizer.*

*Line your baking sheet with aluminum foil or parchment paper
to speed cleanup and prevent sticking.*

SERVES 8 / PREP TIME: 15 MINUTES OR LESS / TOTAL TIME: 1 HOUR AND 30 MINUTES OR LESS

1 large eggplant
1 tablespoon olive oil
1 red onion, chopped
2 garlic cloves, minced
2 tomatoes, seeded and chopped
1 cucumber, peeled, seeded, and
  chopped

1 to 2 tablespoons fresh lemon juice, or
  to taste
1/3 cup chopped fresh Italian parsley
1/4 cup crumbled feta cheese
Salt and freshly ground black pepper

Preheat the oven to 350 degrees. Lightly coat a rimmed baking sheet with nonstick cooking spray.

Lightly coat the eggplant with nonstick cooking spray and place on the baking sheet.

Bake for 50 to 60 minutes, or until very soft. Set aside to cool.

In a large skillet over medium-high heat, add oil. Sauté the onion for 5 to 8 minutes, or until softened. Add garlic, tomatoes, and cucumber and sauté for 3 to 5 minutes, or until the vegetables release their liquids. Set aside to cool.

When eggplant is cool enough to handle, peel and chop. Transfer to a bowl and stir to soften. Add onion mixture and stir well to combine. Add 1 tablespoon lemon juice, parsley, and feta. Season with salt and pepper. Add the remaining lemon juice if desired.

Per Serving	
Calories	75
Calories from Fat	25
Total Fat	3.0 g
Saturated Fat	1.0 g
Trans Fat	0.0 g
Polyunsaturated Fat	0.3 g
Monounsaturated Fat	1.5 g
Cholesterol	5 mg
Sodium	60 mg
Total Carbohydrate	11 g
Dietary Fiber	3 g
Sugars	5 g
Protein	2 g

ROASTED POTATOES AND BABY CARROTS

Both kids and adults who shun veggies seem to make exceptions for roasted red potatoes and baby carrots. A sprinkle of fresh thyme adds a special touch.

Line your baking sheet with aluminum foil or parchment paper to speed cleanup.

SERVES 4 / PREP TIME: 15 MINUTES OR LESS / TOTAL TIME: 45 MINUTES OR LESS

1 tablespoon olive oil
1 (1-pound) bag baby carrots
1 pound small red potatoes, quartered

1 teaspoon fresh thyme leaves
Salt and freshly ground black pepper

Preheat the oven to 400 degrees. Brush a rimmed baking sheet lightly with oil.

Place carrots and potatoes, cut side down, on the baking sheet. Drizzle with oil and sprinkle with thyme, salt, and pepper. Toss to lightly coat.

Roast for 15 minutes, remove from the oven, and stir to combine. Roast for 10 to 15 minutes, or until vegetables are tender and slightly charred.

Roasting potatoes with the skin on provides an extra boost of fiber to your diet.

Per Serving
Calories 160
  Calories from Fat 30
Total Fat . . . . 3.5 g
  Saturated Fat . . . . 0.5 g
  Trans Fat . . . . 0.0 g
  Polyunsaturated Fat . . . . 0.5 g
  Monounsaturated Fat . . . . . . 2.5 g
Cholesterol . . . . 0 mg
Sodium . . . . 80 mg
Total Carbohydrate . . . . 30 g
  Dietary Fiber . . . . 6 g
  Sugars . . . . 5 g
Protein . . . . 4 g

SAUTÉED SPINACH WITH GARLIC

*Spinach shrinks down dramatically during cooking, so don't be alarmed
if it looks like you're cooking for a family of twelve when you start adding the greens.
Cook just until bright green for optimum flavor.*

SERVES 4 / PREP TIME: 15 MINUTES OR LESS / TOTAL TIME: 15 MINUTES OR LESS

1 tablespoon olive oil
3 garlic cloves, minced
1 (9- or 10-ounce) bag baby spinach

In a large skillet over medium-high heat, add oil. Sauté the garlic for 1 minute, or until aromatic and beginning to color. Add spinach and sauté for 1 to 3 minutes, or until bright green and wilted.

Spinach is low in calories, packed with nutrients and easy to prepare—what's not to like?

Per Serving	
Calories	50
Calories from Fat	30
Total Fat	3.5 g
Saturated Fat	0.5 g
Trans Fat	0.0 g
Polyunsaturated Fat	0.4 g
Monounsaturated Fat	2.5 g
Cholesterol	0 mg
Sodium	50 mg
Total Carbohydrate	3 g
Dietary Fiber	1 g
Sugars	0 g
Protein	2 g

ROASTED BRUSSELS SPROUTS

*Roasting at high heat transforms even sturdy, fibrous vegetables
like Brussels sprouts into a tender, deeply flavorful side dish.*

*For a splurge, sprinkle with chopped pancetta, a flavorful Italian bacon,
which permeates the sprouts with a smoky, salty flavor as they roast.
These spiffed-up sprouts are a good example of how a fatty meat,
when used in moderation, can be an acceptable addition to a dish.*

Line your baking sheet with aluminum foil or parchment paper to speed cleanup.

SERVES 4 / PREP TIME: 15 MINUTES OR LESS / TOTAL TIME: 30 MINUTES OR LESS

---

1 ounce pancetta, finely chopped, or
  1 tablespoon olive oil
1 pound Brussels sprouts, trimmed and
  halved lengthwise

3 garlic cloves, thinly sliced
Salt and freshly ground black pepper

Preheat the oven to 400 degrees. Lightly coat a rimmed baking sheet with nonstick cooking spray or brush lightly with oil.

Place Brussels sprouts cut side down on the baking sheet. Sprinkle with pancetta or drizzle with oil and sprinkle with salt and pepper.

Roast for 10 minutes, remove from the oven, and stir well to combine. Roast for 5 to 10 minutes, or until vegetables are tender and slightly charred.

Brussels spouts are a member of the cruciferous vegetable family, which has cancer-fighting properties. Look for sprouts with tight, bright green heads.

Per Serving	
Calories	70
Calories from Fat	25
Total Fat	3.0 g
Saturated Fat	0.8 g
Trans Fat	0.0 g
Polyunsaturated Fat	0.6 g
Monounsaturated Fat	1.2 g
Cholesterol	5 mg
Sodium	155 mg
Total Carbohydrate	11 g
Dietary Fiber	3 g
Sugars	4 g
Protein	4 g

COOK'S NOTES

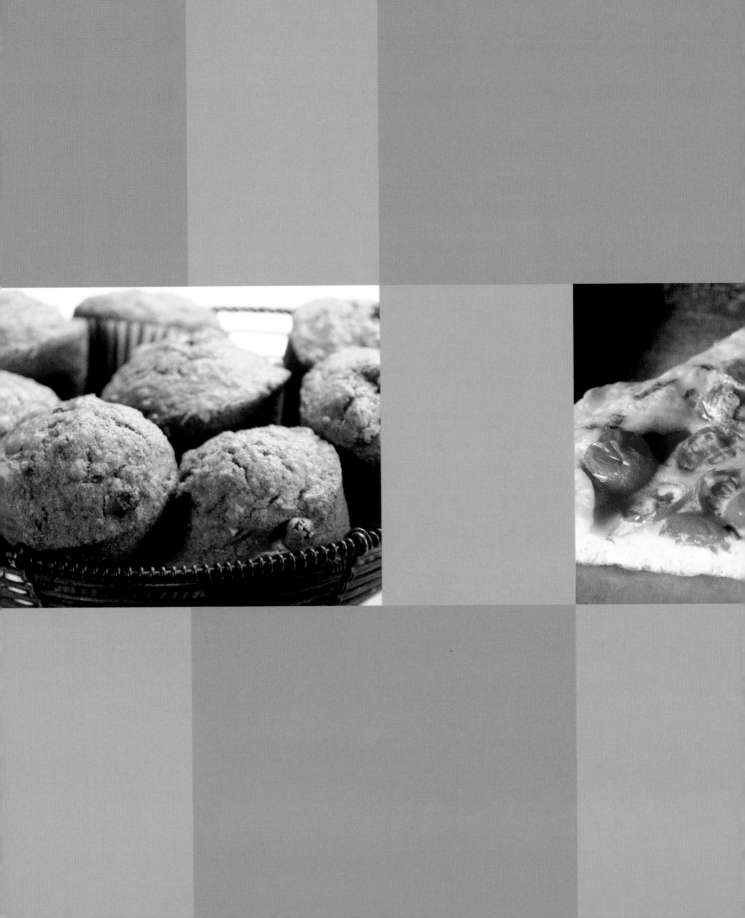

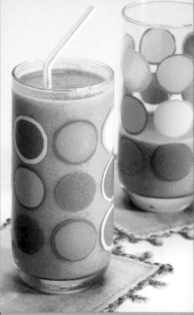

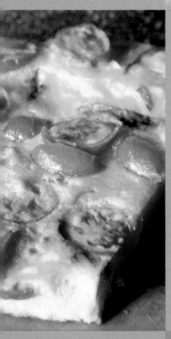

BREAKFAST

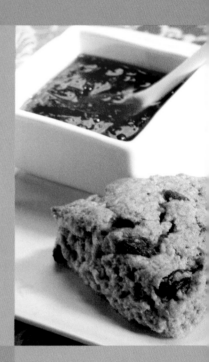

You won't want to hit the snooze button when you see what's in store for breakfast! Flavorful and nutritious, these recipes offer the ultimate wake-up call. Whether you need quick choices for busy weekday mornings, or have time for a more leisurely indulgence on the weekend, your tastebuds will dance with joy as your day gets off to a healthy start.

Another benefit: breakfast eaters tend to eat fewer calories throughout the day, and most people who have successfully lost weight and kept it off say that they eat breakfast on most days of the week.

Now that's a meal worth getting up for!

HAM AND VEGETABLE FRITTATA

This frittata is an impressive brunch dish for entertaining guests, or when served with a salad, it makes a light but satisfying dinner on a busy night.

Reminiscent of the classic "western omelet," this frittata satisfies a ham and cheese craving, but in moderation.

A nonstick pan allows the frittata to be easily removed after cooking and is highly recommended. Make sure to use an oven mitt after removing the pan from the oven.

SERVES 4 / PREP TIME: 15 MINUTES OR LESS / TOTAL TIME: 30 MINUTES OR LESS

---

2 teaspoons canola oil
1/2 cup sliced mushrooms
1/4 cup chopped green or red bell pepper
2 tablespoons finely chopped red onion
8 eggs

2 ounces (about 3 deli slices) ham, cut into thin strips
1 ounce (about 1 deli slice) Swiss cheese, cut into thin strips
Salt and freshly ground black pepper

Preheat the oven to 350 degrees.

In a 10- or 11-inch nonstick, ovenproof skillet over medium-high heat, add oil. Sauté the mushrooms, bell pepper, and onion for 3 to 5 minutes, or until softened.

Meanwhile, in a bowl, beat the eggs. Add ham and cheese and sprinkle with salt and pepper.

Reduce the heat to medium. Pour in egg mixture and cook without stirring for 30 to 45 seconds, or until the eggs are set on the bottom. Continue cooking, using a spatula to lift the edges of the frittata toward the center of the skillet, while gently tilting the pan so the uncooked eggs run underneath the bottom of the frittata. Cook for 15 to 20 seconds, repeating the process several times until the egg on top is still wet, but not runny. Don't worry if the frittata looks a little lumpy.

Transfer to the oven and bake for 3 to 7 minutes, or until the top is just set. Do not overcook. Remove from the oven and let sit for 1 minute. Carefully run a spatula around the skillet edge to loosen the frittata and slide out or invert onto a serving plate.

Per Serving	
Calories	220
Calories from Fat	135
Total Fat	15.0 g
Saturated Fat	4.8 g
Trans Fat	0.1 g
Polyunsaturated Fat	2.2 g
Monounsaturated Fat	6.0 g
Cholesterol	435 mg
Sodium	340 mg
Total Carbohydrate	3 g
Dietary Fiber	0 g
Sugars	1 g
Protein	18 g

BROWN SUGAR YOGURT PARFAIT

Layering yogurt with fresh berries and crunchy granola is a great way to maximize textures in a healthful breakfast or dessert parfait.

Sweetening yogurt to taste saves a lot of the unnecessary sugar found in presweetened yogurts.

The parfait looks very enticing served in a goblet, wine glass, or wide-bottomed tumbler. With a narrow glass, you'll be able to get two layers; if your glass or bowl is wider, just one should do it.

SERVES 1 / PREP TIME: 15 MINUTES OR LESS / TOTAL TIME: 15 MINUTES OR LESS

---

1 (6-ounce) container nonfat plain
   yogurt
2 teaspoons light brown sugar
1/2 cup sliced strawberries or blueberries

1/4 cup Ginger–Cranberry Granola
   (page 148) or purchased granola

In a bowl, combine yogurt and brown sugar.
   In a glass or bowl, decoratively layer berries, yogurt, and granola.

A 1/2 cup of sliced strawberries
has only about 25 calories.

. . . . .

Look for yogurt with live and active cultures.
They are actually "good" bacteria that help
strengthen the immune system.

Per Serving
Calories 250
  Calories from Fat 30
Total Fat . . . . 3.5 g
  Saturated Fat . . . . 0.5 g
  Trans Fat . . . . 0.0 g
  Polyunsaturated Fat . . . . 1.0 g
  Monounsaturated Fat . . . . . . 1.7 g
Cholesterol . . . . 10 mg
Sodium . . . . 120 mg
Total Carbohydrate . . . . 45 g
  Dietary Fiber . . . . 4 g
  Sugars . . . . 31 g
Protein . . . . 12 g

RASPBERRY–PEACH YOGURT SMOOTHIE

This creamy smoothie is a great on-the-go breakfast. Not only that, it's a great way to get calcium and two servings of fruit in a jiffy.

If you prefer a tarter drink, use plain yogurt. For a slightly sweeter drink, add a teaspoon or so of honey or use vanilla yogurt.

SERVES 2 / PREP TIME: 15 MINUTES OR LESS / TOTAL TIME: 15 MINUTES OR LESS

1 cup frozen raspberries
1 cup frozen peaches

1 (6-ounce) container nonfat plain or
 vanilla yogurt
¾ cup apple juice

In a blender, combine raspberries, peaches, yogurt, and juice. Process until smooth.

Frozen fruits are just as nutritious as fresh fruits and, in some cases, even more so. They are a great choice when your favorite fresh fruits are not in season.

Per Serving
Calories 165
 Calories from Fat 5
Total Fat . . . . 0.5 g
 Saturated Fat . . . . 0.1 g
 Trans Fat . . . . 0.0 g
 Polyunsaturated Fat . . . . 0.2 g
 Monounsaturated Fat . . . . . . 0.1 g
Cholesterol . . . . 5 mg
Sodium . . . . 60 mg
Total Carbohydrate . . . . 37 g
 Dietary Fiber . . . . 2 g
 Sugars . . . . 33 g
Protein . . . . 6 g

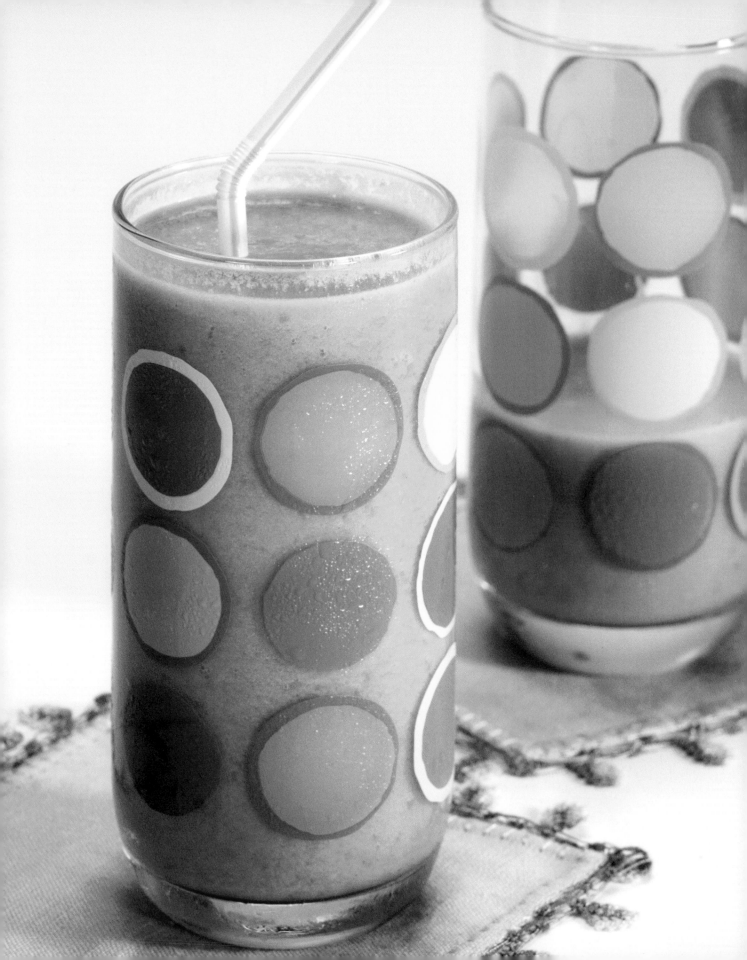

WHOLE GRAIN GINGERBREAD WAFFLES

These aromatic waffles are a breakfast delight. The health benefits of oats, whole wheat flour, and cornmeal are an added bonus. If desired, top with fresh berries.

SERVES 4 / PREP TIME: 30 MINUTES OR LESS / TOTAL TIME: 30 MINUTES OR LESS

1 cup nonfat or low-fat buttermilk
1/4 cup rolled oats
1/3 cup whole wheat flour
1/3 cup all-purpose flour
2 tablespoons cornmeal
1 tablespoon light brown sugar
1 teaspoon ground ginger
1/2 teaspoon ground cinnamon

1/2 teaspoon baking powder
1/2 teaspoon baking soda
1/4 teaspoon salt
Pinch ground cloves
1 egg
1 tablespoon molasses
2 teaspoons canola oil

In a bowl, combine buttermilk and oats. Set aside for 15 minutes.

In a bowl, combine both types of flour, cornmeal, brown sugar, ginger, cinnamon, baking powder, baking soda, salt, and cloves.

In a bowl, beat egg, molasses, and oil. Add to oat mixture. Add wet ingredients to the dry ingredients and stir until just moistened.

Coat a waffle iron with nonstick cooking spray and preheat. Spoon in enough batter to cover 3/4 of the surface. Cook according to waffle iron instructions.

Per Serving	
Calories	200
Calories from Fat	40
Total Fat	4.5 g
Saturated Fat	1.0 g
Trans Fat	0.0 g
Polyunsaturated Fat	1.1 g
Monounsaturated Fat	2.1 g
Cholesterol	55 mg
Sodium	435 mg
Total Carbohydrate	32 g
Dietary Fiber	3 g
Sugars	10 g
Protein	7 g

STRAWBERRY–BANANA SMOOTHIE

*Turn your favorite flavored yogurt into a refreshing drink,
great for breakfast, lunch-on-the-go, or a snack.*

*Even kids who turn up their noses at fresh fruit or plain yogurt
will change their tune when presented with this frosty shake.*

SERVES 2 / PREP TIME: 15 MINUTES OR LESS / TOTAL TIME: 15 MINUTES OR LESS

1 small banana
1 cup frozen strawberries

1 (6-ounce) container nonfat plain or
  vanilla yogurt
$\frac{1}{2}$ cup apple or orange juice

In a blender, combine banana, strawberries, yogurt, and juice. Process until smooth.

Smoothies are a delicious and easy way
to add more fruits to your day.

Per Serving
Calories 140
  Calories from Fat 0
Total Fat . . . . 0.0 g
  Saturated Fat . . . . 0.2 g
  Trans Fat . . . . 0.0 g
  Polyunsaturated Fat . . . . 0.1 g
  Monounsaturated Fat . . . . . . 0.1 g
Cholesterol . . . . 5 mg
Sodium . . . . 60 mg
Total Carbohydrate . . . . 32 g
  Dietary Fiber . . . . 3 g
  Sugars . . . . 22 g
Protein . . . . 5 g

PUMPKIN-SPICE PANCAKES

Add nutrients and variety to breakfast by adding puréed fruit or vegetables to store-bought pancake mix. Canned pumpkin purée is one of the easiest ways to sneak in a healthy dose of vitamin A, as well as potassium, fiber, and flavor.

The inside of these pancakes will take a little longer to cook through than regular pancakes, so it might be necessary to turn down the heat to avoid overcooking the outside before the inside is done.

Since cooking directions for each brand of pancake mix can vary slightly, prepare pancakes according to the directions for 1 cup of mix before adding the pumpkin and spices.

SERVES 4 / PREP TIME: 15 MINUTES OR LESS / TOTAL TIME: 30 MINUTES OR LESS

---

1 egg
1 cup baking or pancake mix, such as Bisquick
1/2 cup plus 2 tablespoons low-fat (1%) milk
1/2 cup canned pumpkin

1/4 cup chopped pecans, optional
1 tablespoon light brown sugar
1/2 teaspoon ground ginger
1/4 teaspoon ground cinnamon
Pinch ground cloves
Pinch ground nutmeg

In a bowl, beat egg. Add baking mix, milk, pumpkin, pecans, brown sugar, ginger, cinnamon, cloves, and nutmeg.

Lightly coat a nonstick skillet or griddle with nonstick cooking spray and heat to medium. When a drop of water sizzles when it hits the pan, it's ready. Pour 1/4 cup of batter into the skillet for each pancake. When the bottom is golden, turn over and cook the other side. Reduce the heat to medium-low and cook until insides are cooked through and pancakes bounce back when touched.

Pumpkin is filled with beta-carotene, which may protect against cancers and heart disease. Canned pumpkin is almost equal to fresh in nutrients.

Per Serving	
Calories	190
Calories from Fat	55
Total Fat	6.0 g
Saturated Fat	1.9 g
Trans Fat	1.2 g
Polyunsaturated Fat	1.4 g
Monounsaturated Fat	1.8 g
Cholesterol	55 mg
Sodium	430 mg
Total Carbohydrate	29 g
Dietary Fiber	2 g
Sugars	7 g
Protein	6 g

BUTTERMILK BRAN MUFFINS

Fiber is an important part of a healthy diet. These bran muffins are hearty without being heavy. Made with bran cereal, they take only a few minutes to whip up. You can add other dried fruit or nuts or omit the raisins.

MAKES 12 MUFFINS / PREP TIME: 15 MINUTES OR LESS / TOTAL TIME: 45 MINUTES OR LESS

1/2 cup boiling water
1 1/2 cups 100% bran cereal, such as
   All-Bran (not flakes)
1 egg
1 cup buttermilk
1/4 cup canola oil
1 1/4 cups all-purpose flour

1/2 cup light brown sugar
1 1/4 teaspoons baking soda
1/2 teaspoon ground cinnamon
1/4 teaspoon salt
1 cup finely chopped dried fruit, such
   as Sun-Maid Fruit Bits, or raisins

Preheat the oven to 375 degrees. Lightly coat a muffin tin with nonstick cooking spray or fill with paper liners.

In a heatproof bowl, pour water over bran and stir to combine.

In a bowl, beat egg. Add buttermilk and oil and stir to combine. Add bran mixture, flour, brown sugar, baking soda, cinnamon, and salt and stir until just combined. Add dried fruit and stir gently to incorporate. Spoon batter evenly into muffin cups.

Bake for 18 to 23 minutes, or until tops just bounce back when touched. Leave in tins for 5 minutes before removing to a cooling rack.

These muffins are great for breakfast or a mid-afternoon snack.

Per Serving	
Calories	195
Calories from Fat	55
Total Fat	6.0 g
Saturated Fat	0.6 g
Trans Fat	0.0 g
Polyunsaturated Fat	1.6 g
Monounsaturated Fat	3.0 g
Cholesterol	20 mg
Sodium	235 mg
Total Carbohydrate	35 g
Dietary Fiber	4 g
Sugars	19 g
Protein	4 g

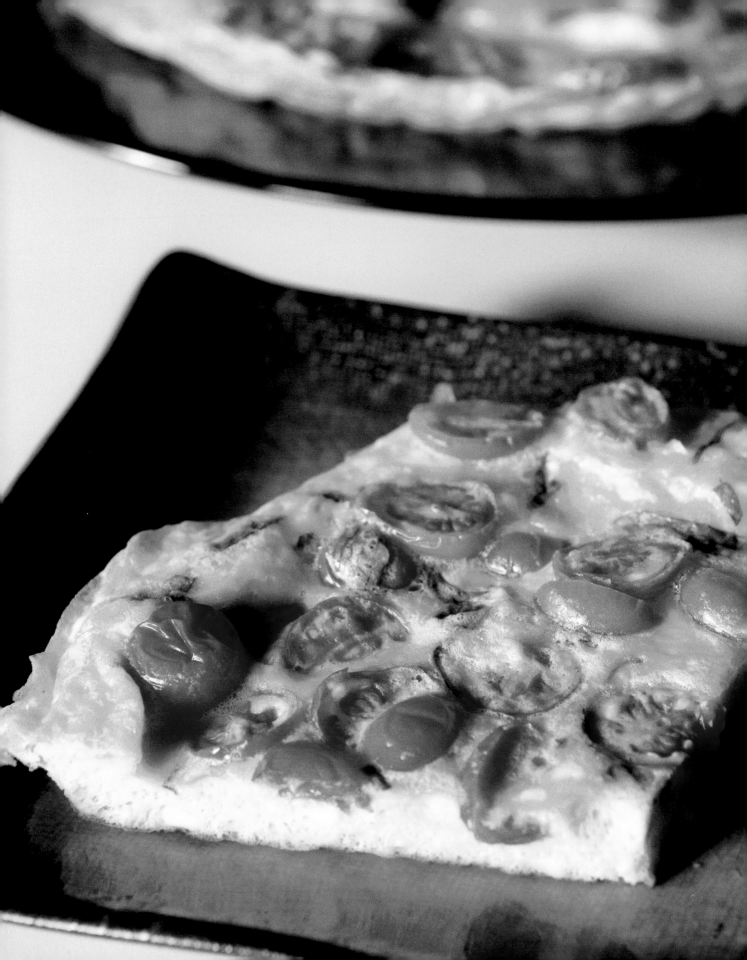

TOMATO AND BASIL FRITTATA

For a cook, summer has long been synonymous with fresh and abundant tomatoes and basil. These days, however, with fresh herbs and flavorful grape tomatoes available year-round, this dynamic duo can be enjoyed all year long.

Frittatas, oven-baked omelets, are not only a welcome breakfast, but are ideal for a simple dinner or lunch.

A nonstick pan allows the frittata to be easily removed after cooking and is highly recommended. If you don't have a reliable ovenproof nonstick pan, make sure to oil the pan before adding the eggs.

Make sure to use an oven mitt after removing the pan from the oven.

SERVES 4 / PREP TIME: 15 MINUTES OR LESS / TOTAL TIME: 30 MINUTES OR LESS

---

8 eggs
1 cup halved grape tomatoes
1/4 cup coarsely chopped fresh basil

1/3 cup crumbled feta cheese
Salt and freshly ground black pepper

Preheat the oven to 350 degrees.

In a bowl, beat the eggs. Gently add tomatoes, basil, and feta and sprinkle with salt and pepper.

Coat a 10- or 11-inch nonstick, ovenproof skillet with nonstick cooking spray and place over medium heat. Pour in egg mixture and cook without stirring for 30 to 45 seconds, or until the eggs are set on the bottom. Continue cooking, using a spatula to lift the edges of the frittata toward the center of the skillet, while gently tilting the pan so the uncooked eggs run underneath the bottom of the frittata. Cook for 15 to 20 seconds, repeating the process several times until the egg on top is still wet, but not runny. Don't worry if the frittata looks a little lumpy.

Transfer to the oven and bake for 3 to 7 minutes, or until the top is just set. Do not overcook. Remove from the oven and let sit for 1 minute. Carefully run a spatula around the skillet edge to loosen the frittata and slide out or invert onto a serving plate.

Per Serving	
Calories	185
Calories from Fat	115
Total Fat	13.0 g
Saturated Fat	5.0 g
Trans Fat	0.1 g
Polyunsaturated Fat	1.5 g
Monounsaturated Fat	4.4 g
Cholesterol	435 mg
Sodium	280 mg
Total Carbohydrate	3 g
Dietary Fiber	1 g
Sugars	2 g
Protein	15 g

BAKED EGGS FLORENTINE

A baked egg dish is an elegant way to start your day or delight breakfast guests.
If you like your eggs well done, use standard eggs.
If you like your eggs softer, choose pasteurized whole eggs.

SERVES 4 / PREP TIME: 15 MINUTES OR LESS / TOTAL TIME: 30 MINUTES OR LESS

2 tablespoons Italian–style bread crumbs
2 tablespoons freshly grated Parmesan
  cheese
1 tablespoon olive oil
1 (9- or 10-ounce) bag baby spinach

4 eggs
Salt and freshly ground black pepper
2 whole wheat English muffins, split
  and toasted

Preheat the oven to 300 degrees.

In a bowl, combine bread crumbs and cheese.

In a 10-inch ovenproof skillet over medium-high heat, add oil. Sauté the spinach until bright green and wilted. Remove from heat and spread spinach over the bottom of the skillet. Carefully crack eggs, one at a time, over spinach, spacing them evenly in the pan. Sprinkle with salt, pepper, bread crumbs, and cheese.

Transfer to the oven and bake for 8 to 12 minutes, or until the eggs are cooked to desired firmness. With a spatula, carefully scoop up an egg and spinach and set on top of English muffin half.

Per Serving	
Calories	210
Calories from Fat	90
Total Fat	10.0 g
Saturated Fat	2.6 g
Trans Fat	0.0 g
Polyunsaturated Fat	1.5 g
Monounsaturated Fat	5.0 g
Cholesterol	215 mg
Sodium	310 mg
Total Carbohydrate	18 g
Dietary Fiber	3 g
Sugars	3 g
Protein	12 g

BANANA PANCAKES

There's no better way to face the morning than with these banana pancakes made with whole wheat flour and oats. They are a perfect example of how healthy and tasty can go hand-in-hand.

SERVES 5 / PREP TIME: 15 MINUTES OR LESS / TOTAL TIME: 30 MINUTES OR LESS

¾ cup all-purpose flour

½ cup whole wheat flour

¼ cup rolled oats

2 tablespoons granulated sugar

2 teaspoons baking powder

½ teaspoon salt

2 ripe bananas, divided

2 eggs, beaten

1 cup low-fat (1%) milk

3 tablespoons canola oil

In a bowl, combine both types of flour, oats, sugar, baking powder, and salt.

In a bowl, mash one banana (a big fork or potato masher works well). Add eggs and stir to combine. Add milk and oil and stir to combine. Add liquid mixture to the flour mixture and stir gently until just combined. Cut the remaining banana into thin slices.

Lightly coat a nonstick skillet or griddle with nonstick cooking spray and heat to medium. When a drop of water sizzles when it hits the pan, it's ready. Pour ¼ cup of batter into the skillet for each pancake. Cook until bubbles appear on top. Press 3 to 4 slices of banana into each pancake. When the bottom is golden, turn over and cook until insides are cooked through and pancakes bounce back when touched.

Per Serving	
Calories	315
Calories from Fat	110
Total Fat	12 g
Saturated Fat	1.7 g
Trans Fat	0.0 g
Polyunsaturated Fat	3.1 g
Monounsaturated Fat	6.0 g
Cholesterol	90 mg
Sodium	430 mg
Total Carbohydrate	45 g
Dietary Fiber	4 g
Sugars	14 g
Protein	9 g

CARROT–APPLESAUCE MUFFINS

These delicious muffins are infused with autumnal spices, like cinnamon, cardamom, and ginger. Shredded carrots and coconut add texture. Using applesauce instead of extra oil keeps the muffins moist and lower in calories.

MAKES 12 MUFFINS / PREP TIME: 15 MINUTES OR LESS / TOTAL TIME: 45 MINUTES OR LESS

1¼ cups all-purpose flour
¾ cup whole wheat flour
¾ cup light brown sugar
1½ teaspoons baking soda
1 teaspoon ground cardamom
1 teaspoon ground ginger
½ teaspoon ground cinnamon
½ teaspoon salt

1½ cups grated carrots
½ cup raisins
½ cup sweetened shredded coconut
½ cup chopped pecans, optional
2 eggs
½ cup canola oil
1 cup unsweetened applesauce

Preheat the oven to 350 degrees. Lightly coat a muffin tin with nonstick cooking spray or fill with paper liners.

In a bowl, combine both types of flour, sugar, baking soda, cardamom, ginger, cinnamon, and salt. Stir in carrots, raisins, coconut, and pecans.

In a bowl, beat eggs. Add oil and applesauce and stir until well combined. Add to flour mixture and stir until just combined. Spoon batter evenly into muffin cups.

Bake for 25 to 30 minutes, or until tops just bounce back when touched. Leave in tins for 5 minutes before removing to a cooling rack.

Per Serving	
Calories	265
Calories from Fat	100
Total Fat	11.0 g
Saturated Fat	1.8 g
Trans Fat	0.0 g
Polyunsaturated Fat	3.0 g
Monounsaturated Fat	5.7 g
Cholesterol	35 mg
Sodium	290 mg
Total Carbohydrate	39 g
Dietary Fiber	2 g
Sugars	21 g
Protein	4 g

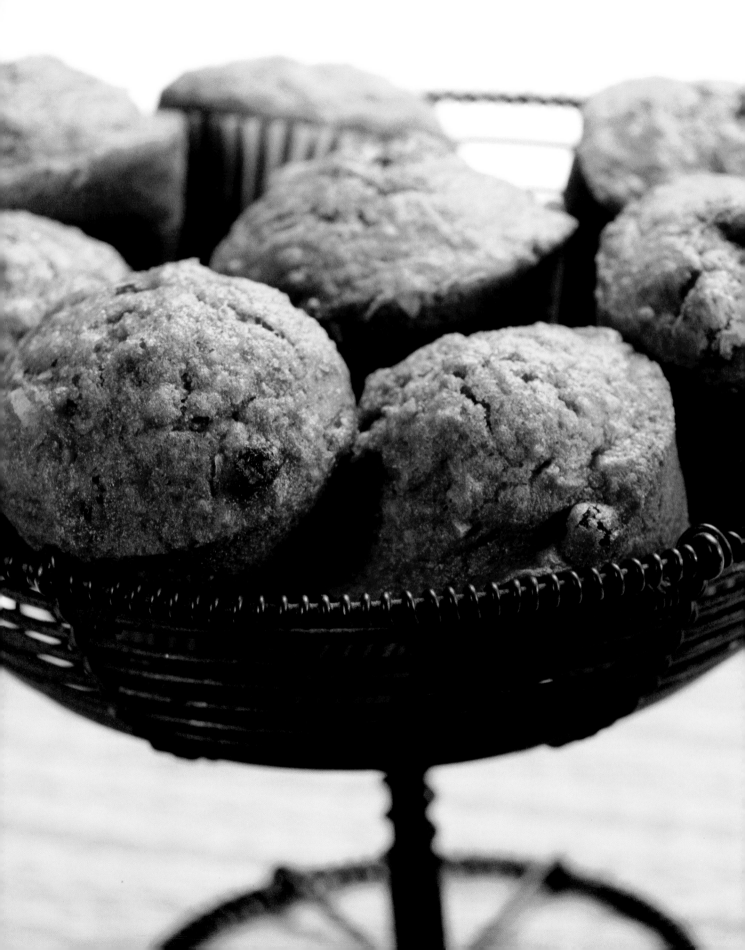

FRUITY MORNING OATMEAL

Whether you like your oatmeal sweetened or "as is," everyone can agree that fortifying your bowl with fresh or dried fruit to add texture and flavor is welcome.

If you're a member of the sweet camp, sprinkle with a bit of brown sugar.

SERVES 2 / PREP TIME: 15 MINUTES OR LESS / TOTAL TIME: 15 MINUTES OR LESS

1³/₄ cups low-fat (1%) or skim milk
¹/₈ teaspoon salt
1 cup old-fashioned rolled oats
  (not quick cooking)

1 apple, peeled, cored, and chopped
¹/₄ cup dried and sweetened cranberries,
  such as Craisins, or raisins
1 teaspoon light brown sugar, optional

In a saucepan, combine milk and salt and bring to a boil. Reduce the heat to medium, stir in oats, apple, cranberries, and brown sugar, and cook, stirring occasionally, until thickened.

Oatmeal has many heart-healthy benefits. It is low in saturated fat and sodium and is full of iron, magnesium, and soluble fiber, which helps lower cholesterol.

Per Serving	
Calories	335
Calories from Fat	45
Total Fat	5.0 g
Saturated Fat	1.8 g
Trans Fat	0.0 g
Polyunsaturated Fat	1.1 g
Monounsaturated Fat	1.4 g
Cholesterol	15 mg
Sodium	260 mg
Total Carbohydrate	60 g
Dietary Fiber	6 g
Sugars	29 g
Protein	14 g

DRIED FRUIT COMPOTE

Compote (stewed fruit) can be served on its own or as a topping for oatmeal or yogurt for breakfast or dessert. A little goes a long way toward providing sweetness and adding texture.

SERVES 6 / PREP TIME: 15 MINUTES OR LESS / TOTAL TIME: 15 MINUTES OR LESS

½ cup dried apricots, quartered

½ cup dried pitted prunes, quartered

½ cup finely chopped dried fruit, such as Sun-Maid Fruit Bits, or raisins

¼ cup dried and sweetened cranberries, such as Craisins

1 cup apple juice

6 cloves

1 cinnamon stick

In a saucepan, combine apricots, prunes, fruit bits, cranberries, apple juice, cloves, and cinnamon and bring to a boil, stirring to combine. Reduce the heat and simmer for 8 to 10 minutes, or until juice is absorbed, stirring occasionally. Let cool and discard cloves and cinnamon stick.

Prunes—also known as dried plums—are high in fiber and potassium. Apricots are power-packed with beta-carotene and other disease-fighting antioxidants.

Per Serving	
Calories	140
Calories from Fat	0
Total Fat	0.0 g
Saturated Fat	0.0 g
Trans Fat	0.0 g
Polyunsaturated Fat	0.1 g
Monounsaturated Fat	0.1 g
Cholesterol	0 mg
Sodium	10 mg
Total Carbohydrate	35 g
Dietary Fiber	3 g
Sugars	28 g
Protein	1 g

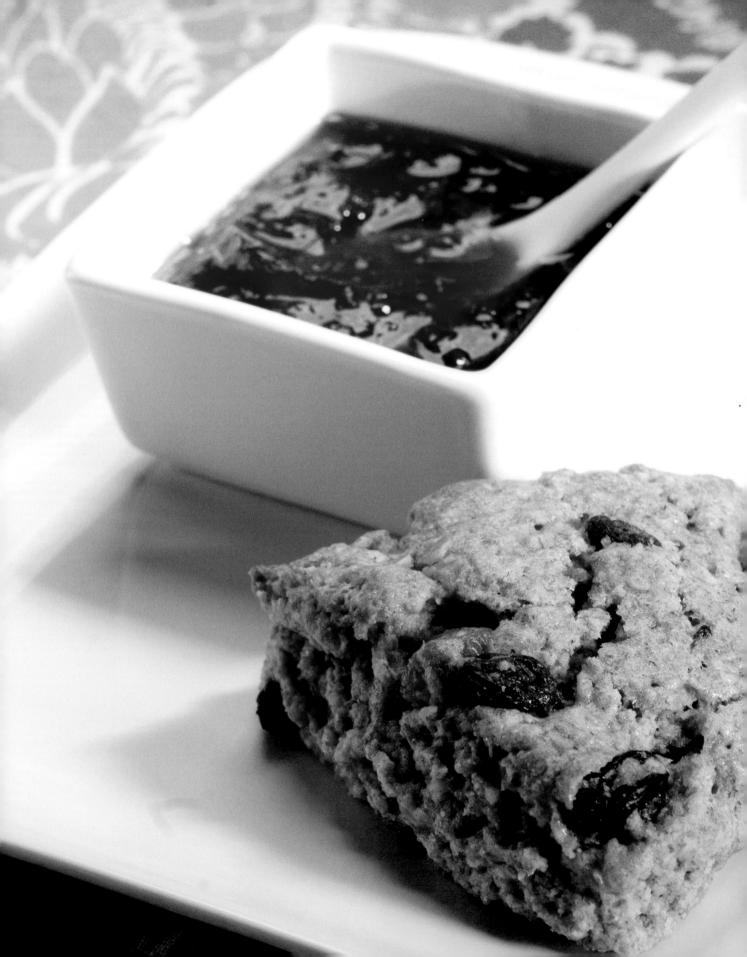

OATMEAL–RAISIN SCONES

While whole wheat scones can be leaden and heavy,
this oatmeal version is light, airy, and studded with raisins.

Mixing in a food processor speeds the prep and keeps the dough
from becoming overworked. To ensure the scones remain tender,
use caution not to overbake. Using insulated baking sheets or
double stacking sheets prevents the bottoms from overbrowning.

For added flavor, add the zest from an orange.

MAKES 12 SCONES / PREP TIME: 15 MINUTES OR LESS / TOTAL TIME: 30 MINUTES OR LESS

1¾ cups whole wheat flour
1½ cups rolled oats
⅓ cup granulated sugar
½ teaspoon baking soda
2 teaspoons baking powder
½ teaspoon salt

½ cup (1 stick) butter, chilled and cut
  into pieces
¾ cup buttermilk
1 cup raisins, preferably a mix of
  regular and golden
1 egg, beaten

Preheat the oven to 400 degrees. Line a baking sheet with parchment paper or lightly coat with nonstick cooking spray.

In a food processor, pulse flour, oats, sugar, baking soda, baking powder, and salt to combine.

Add butter and pulse until mixture resembles coarse crumbs. Add buttermilk and pulse until just combined and evenly moistened. Do not allow the dough to form a ball.

Transfer to a bowl and gently knead in raisins. Do not overmix.

Divide dough into three balls. Flatten each ball slightly and cut into four wedges. Place wedges on the baking sheet, leaving 2 inches between scones, and brush lightly with egg. Bake for 13 to 18 minutes, or until golden and firm. Leave for 2 minutes before removing to a cooling rack.

Per Serving	
Calories	235
Calories from Fat	80
Total Fat	9.0 g
Saturated Fat	5.2 g
Trans Fat	0.0 g
Polyunsaturated Fat	0.7 g
Monounsaturated Fat	2.4 g
Cholesterol	40 mg
Sodium	290 mg
Total Carbohydrate	35 g
Dietary Fiber	4 g
Sugars	14 g
Protein	6 g

GINGER–CRANBERRY GRANOLA

*Granola is considered a "health food" by most people and for good reason.
Its combination of whole grains, toasted nuts, and dried fruit
provides nutrients and fiber. Unfortunately, most commercial granolas
are also loaded with added sugar and fat. This homemade version
uses maple syrup for sweetening and only a small amount of oil.*

Serve over yogurt or mix with milk.

*Line your baking sheet with aluminum foil or parchment paper
to speed cleanup and prevent sticking.*

SERVES 12 / PREP TIME: 15 MINUTES OR LESS / TOTAL TIME: 45 MINUTES OR LESS

---

4 cups rolled oats
1/2 cup sliced almonds
1/4 cup unprocessed wheat bran or
    wheat germ
2 teaspoons ground ginger
1/3 cup maple syrup
2 tablespoons canola oil

1 teaspoon vanilla
1/2 cup golden raisins
1/2 cup dried and sweetened cranberries,
    such as Craisins
2 tablespoons chopped crystallized
    ginger

Preheat the oven to 325 degrees.

On a rimmed baking sheet, combine oats, almonds, bran, and ground ginger.

In a bowl, combine maple syrup, oil, and vanilla. Pour over the oat mixture and stir well to moisten.

Bake for 10 minutes. Remove from the oven and stir the mixture thoroughly. Bake for 10 minutes, stirring halfway through. Remove from the oven and stir in the raisins, cranberries, and crystallized ginger. Bake for 5 minutes. Remove the pan from the oven and stir. Cool for 5 minutes and stir again.

Per Serving	
Calories	215
Calories from Fat	55
Total Fat	6.0 g
Saturated Fat	0.6 g
Trans Fat	0.0 g
Polyunsaturated Fat	1.8 g
Monounsaturated Fat	3.1 g
Cholesterol	0 mg
Sodium	0 mg
Total Carbohydrate	36 g
Dietary Fiber	4 g
Sugars	15 g
Protein	6 g

Store nuts in the freezer to preserve freshness.

BLUEBERRY–PEACH–POMEGRANATE SMOOTHIE

Think of this drink as an antioxidant superpower in which blueberries and pomegranate juice unite to fight free radicals.

Many brands of pomegranate juice are now available in several blended flavors. The blueberry blend goes great in this smoothie. If you can't find it, use the plain pomegranate or substitute a cranberry–blueberry juice blend.

SERVES 2 / PREP TIME: 15 MINUTES OR LESS / TOTAL TIME: 15 MINUTES OR LESS

1 cup frozen blueberries
1 cup nonfat vanilla yogurt

1 cup pomegranate or pomegranate–blueberry juice
1/2 cup frozen peaches

In a blender, combine blueberries, yogurt, juice, and peaches. Process until smooth.

Per Serving	
Calories	180
Calories from Fat	5
Total Fat	0.5 g
Saturated Fat	0.1 g
Trans Fat	0.0 g
Polyunsaturated Fat	0.3 g
Monounsaturated Fat	0.1 g
Cholesterol	5 mg
Sodium	70 mg
Total Carbohydrate	41 g
Dietary Fiber	3 g
Sugars	32 g
Protein	4 g

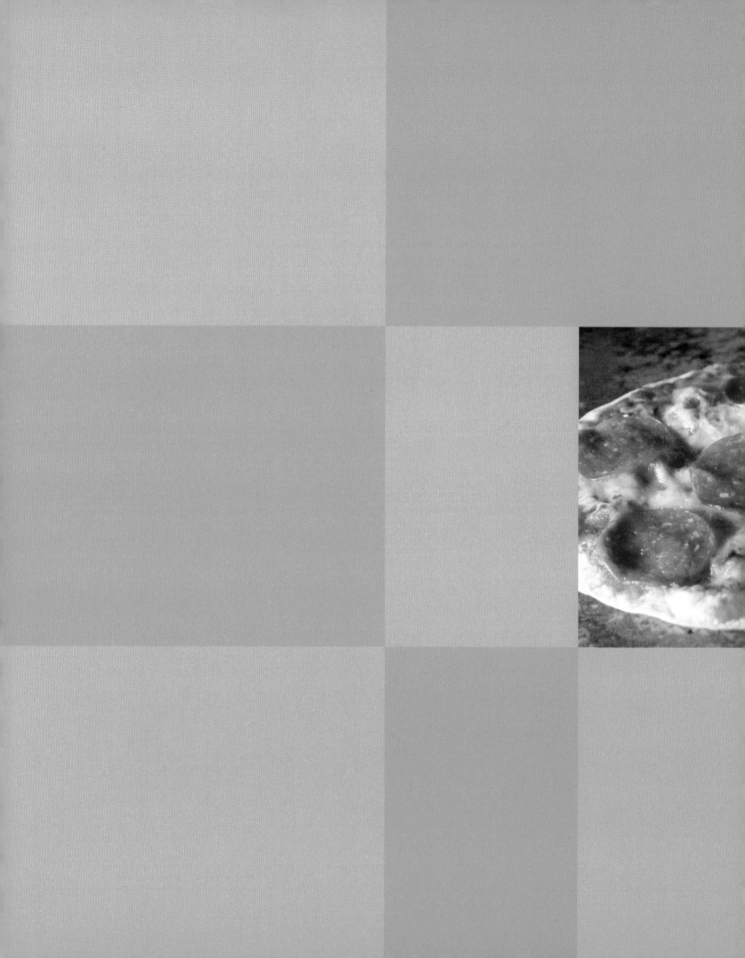

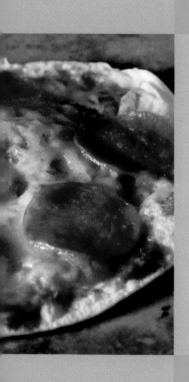

SNACKS

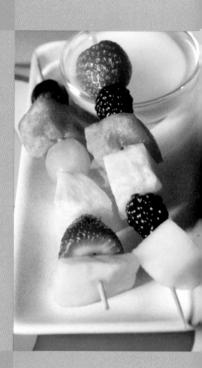

Snacking your way to better health is easy with the right choices. Fruits, vegetables, and whole grains are easy to combine into simple yet satisfying creations for those between-meal times when you just need a little something. Sweet or salty, crunchy or chewy, these snacks will hit the spot whatever you're craving—and hold you over until mealtime.

CHEESY PITA CRISPS

Inevitably, there are always one or two extra pitas after sandwich making. Toasting them with cheese makes a great snack or last-minute appetizer. They are delicious on their own or accompanied by Eggplant Spread (page 123) or a favorite dip.

Top with any shredded or grated hard cheese or the crumbly remnants of a container of feta cheese.

The best way to oil the pitas is to dab them with a pastry brush. Otherwise, drizzle the oil and spread it with the back of a spoon.

SERVES 4 / PREP TIME: 15 MINUTES OR LESS / TOTAL TIME: 15 MINUTES OR LESS

2 (6- to 7-inch) whole wheat pitas
2 teaspoons olive oil

1 tablespoon freshly grated Parmesan
or other cheese

Preheat the oven to 400 degrees.

Split pitas into halves. Using a pastry brush, dab pita halves with oil. Stack and cut into sixths and place wedges, rough side up, on a baking sheet. Sprinkle with cheese.

Bake for 5 to 10 minutes, or until crisp.

Per Serving	
Calories	95
Calories from Fat	30
Total Fat	3.5 g
Saturated Fat	0.6 g
Trans Fat	0.0 g
Polyunsaturated Fat	0.6 g
Monounsaturated Fat	1.9 g
Cholesterol	0 mg
Sodium	75 mg
Total Carbohydrate	15 g
Dietary Fiber	1 g
Sugars	1 g
Protein	3 g

ROSEMARY POPCORN

*Rosemary–infused olive oil adds an adult touch
to the kid-friendly treat, popcorn.*

SERVES 2 / PREP TIME: 15 MINUTES OR LESS / TOTAL TIME: 15 MINUTES OR LESS

1 tablespoon chopped fresh rosemary,
   pounded to bruise
2 tablespoons olive oil

8 cups hot air-popped popcorn (about
   4 tablespoons unpopped)
Salt

In a microwave-safe bowl, microwave oil and rosemary on 50% power for 2 minutes. Set aside. Briefly cool and strain into a bowl.

While popcorn is hot, drizzle with rosemary oil and sprinkle with salt. Toss well to combine.

Use the homemade rosemary oil to flavor Oven–Baked Potato Chips (page 104).

Per Serving	
Calories	245
Calories from Fat	135
Total Fat	15.0 g
Saturated Fat	2.0 g
Trans Fat	0.0 g
Polyunsaturated Fat	2.0 g
Monounsaturated Fat	10.3 g
Cholesterol	0 mg
Sodium	0 mg
Total Carbohydrate	25 g
Dietary Fiber	5 g
Sugars	0 g
Protein	4 g

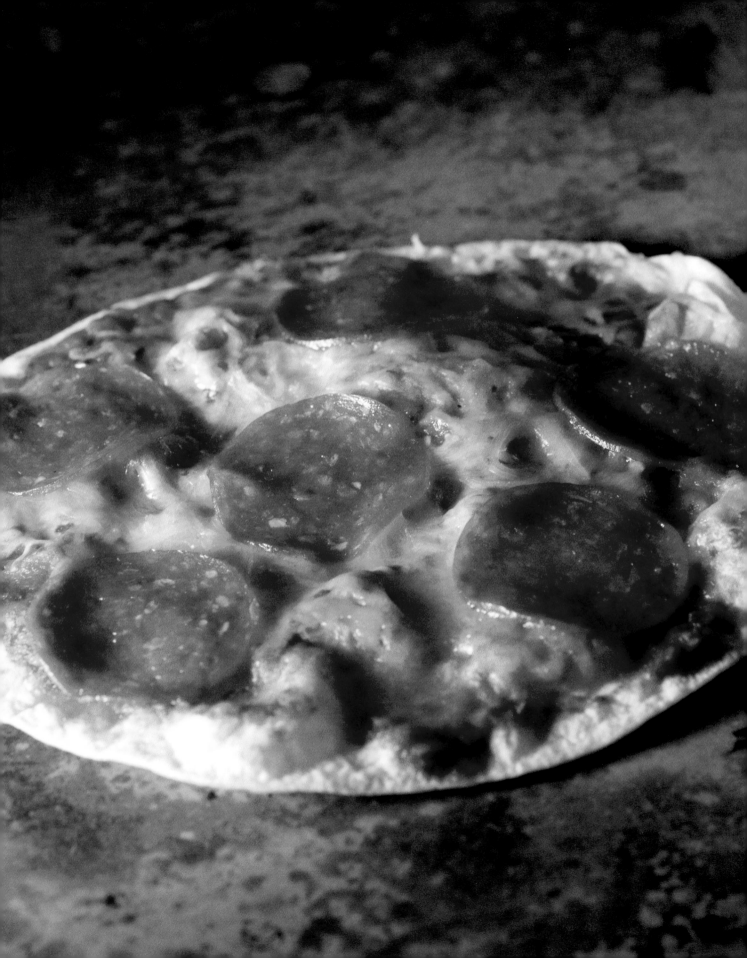

PEPPERONI TORTILLA PIZZA

When you need a pizza fix, try this tortilla version. With fewer calories and less fat than its traditional counterpart, it's the perfect way to satisfy your pepperoni craving without going overboard.

Because each microwave has slightly different power, cooking times can vary slightly. Always start with less and add more if needed.

SERVES 1 / PREP TIME: 15 MINUTES OR LESS / TOTAL TIME: 15 MINUTES OR LESS

---

1 (8-inch) whole wheat or flour tortilla
2 tablespoons pizza sauce
2 tablespoons shredded part-skim mozzarella cheese

1 tablespoon freshly grated Parmesan cheese or a Parmesan blend
6 pepperoni slices

Pierce tortilla in several places with a fork. Place between two sheets of paper towels. Microwave on HIGH for 1 to 1½ minutes, or until barely crisp. Remove from paper towels and place on a microwave-safe plate. Spread with sauce and sprinkle with both cheeses. Top with pepperoni. Microwave on HIGH for 45 seconds, or until cheeses melt.

Tortillas can burn in the microwave if cooked too long. Don't leave unattended.

Per Serving	
Calories	255
Calories from Fat	110
Total Fat	12.0 g
Saturated Fat	4.9 g
Trans Fat	0.0 g
Polyunsaturated Fat	1.9 g
Monounsaturated Fat	4.9 g
Cholesterol	25 mg
Sodium	775 mg
Total Carbohydrate	23 g
Dietary Fiber	4 g
Sugars	3 g
Protein	12 g

CHILI-SPICED POPCORN

Popcorn doesn't have to be laden with butter to taste good.
Here, a drizzle of heart–healthy olive oil and taco spices give it punch.

SERVES 2 / PREP TIME: 15 MINUTES OR LESS / TOTAL TIME: 15 MINUTES OR LESS

¹/₂ teaspoon paprika
¹/₂ teaspoon ground cumin
¹/₂ teaspoon chili powder
¹/₄ teaspoon garlic powder
¹/₄ teaspoon salt

Pinch cayenne pepper
2 tablespoons olive oil
8 cups hot air-popped popcorn (about
  4 tablespoons unpopped)

In a bowl, combine paprika, cumin, chili powder, garlic powder, salt, and cayenne pepper. While popcorn is hot, drizzle with oil and sprinkle with spice mixture. Toss well to combine.

Popcorn is a whole grain—who knew?
Pop some as a snack, but hold the butter
to reduce saturated fat.

Per Serving	
Calories	250
Calories from Fat	135
Total Fat	15.0 g
Saturated Fat	2.0 g
Trans Fat	0.0 g
Polyunsaturated Fat	2.1 g
Monounsaturated Fat	10.4 g
Cholesterol	0 mg
Sodium	315 mg
Total Carbohydrate	26 g
Dietary Fiber	5 g
Sugars	1 g
Protein	4 g

VEGGIE TORTILLA PIZZA

*For a quick snack or light meal, it doesn't get any easier than a tortilla pizza.
A crunchy crust and gooey toppings in under 3 minutes!*

*Because each microwave has slightly different power,
cooking times can vary slightly. Always start with less and add more if needed.*

SERVES 1 / PREP TIME: 15 MINUTES OR LESS / TOTAL TIME: 15 MINUTES OR LESS

1 (8-inch) whole wheat or flour tortilla
2 tablespoons pizza sauce
2 tablespoons shredded part-skim
  mozzarella cheese

1 tablespoon freshly grated Parmesan
  cheese or a Parmesan blend
1/4 cup chopped green or red bell pepper
3 mushrooms, sliced
1 tablespoon chopped red onion

Pierce tortilla in several places with a fork. Place between two sheets of paper towels. Microwave on HIGH for 1 to 1½ minutes, or until barely crisp. Remove from paper towels and place on a microwave-safe plate. Spread with sauce and sprinkle with both cheeses. Top with bell pepper, mushrooms, and onion. Microwave on HIGH for 45 seconds, or until cheeses melt.

Tortillas can burn in the microwave if cooked
too long. Don't leave unattended.

Per Serving	
Calories	220
Calories from Fat	65
Total Fat	7 g
Saturated Fat	2.8 g
Trans Fat	0.0 g
Polyunsaturated Fat	1.5 g
Monounsaturated Fat	2.3 g
Cholesterol	15 mg
Sodium	535 mg
Total Carbohydrate	28 g
Dietary Fiber	5 g
Sugars	5 g
Protein	11 g

CREAMY PEANUT BUTTER DIP

Nothing balances the crunch of an apple or a piece of celery better than a creamy dip. Using peanut butter is a good way to pair protein with carbohydrates for extra energy.

For a real treat, spread over a sliced banana and top with raisins or shredded coconut.

SERVES 4 / PREP TIME: 15 MINUTES OR LESS / TOTAL TIME: 15 MINUTES OR LESS

¼ cup all-natural creamy peanut butter
2 tablespoons nonfat plain or vanilla yogurt
2 teaspoons honey

Pinch cinnamon, optional
Cut-up apples, banana, celery, or other dippers

In a bowl, combine peanut butter, yogurt, honey, and cinnamon until smooth. Serve with fruit or vegetables.

Make sure to use an all-natural peanut butter with no added sugar or additives. In addition to having true peanut flavor, by using "natural" peanut butter you will avoid trans fats and added sugar. Simply mix in the layer of oil on top.

. . . . .

This dip is a delicious way to get more fruit or vegetables into your child's day.

Per Serving
Calories 110
  Calories from Fat 70
Total Fat . . . . 8.0 g
  Saturated Fat . . . . 1.0 g
  Trans Fat . . . . 0.0 g
  Polyunsaturated Fat . . . . 2.0 g
  Monounsaturated Fat . . . . . . 4.0 g
Cholesterol . . . . 0 mg
Sodium . . . . 65 mg
Total Carbohydrate . . . . 6 g
  Dietary Fiber . . . . 1 g
  Sugars . . . . 4 g
Protein . . . . 4 g

MEDITERRANEAN TUNA PÂTÉ

When you need a party spread, you don't have to opt for a high-calorie pâté. This tuna topping, flavored with balsamic vinegar and capers, provides lots of flavor without a lot of fat.

SERVES 12 / PREP TIME: 30 MINUTES OR LESS / TOTAL TIME: 30 MINUTES OR LESS

1 (6-ounce) can white tuna packed in water, drained

3 cups loosely packed cubed, crustless baguette

2 tablespoons balsamic vinegar

2 tablespoons capers, drained

1 hard-boiled egg, roughly chopped

1/4 cup roughly chopped dill pickles (not dill relish)

Juice of 1/2 lemon

1 tablespoon extra–virgin olive oil

Salt and freshly ground black pepper

In a food processor, combine tuna, bread, vinegar, capers, egg, pickles, and lemon juice. Drizzle in the oil and pulse until smooth. Season with salt and pepper.

Capers are the sun-dried unopened flower buds of a Mediterranean bush, "Capparis Spinosa." While some capers are the size of small olives, the most prized ones, the tiny "nonpareil" capers, are about 1/4-inch in diameter. Capers are a wonderful addition to pasta sauces and are often served as a topping for smoked fish.

Per Serving	
Calories	60
Calories from Fat	20
Total Fat	2.0 g
Saturated Fat	0.4 g
Trans Fat	0.0 g
Polyunsaturated Fat	0.3 g
Monounsaturated Fat	1.1 g
Cholesterol	20 mg
Sodium	185 mg
Total Carbohydrate	5 g
Dietary Fiber	0 g
Sugars	1 g
Protein	5 g

FRUIT SKEWERS WITH YOGURT DIPPING SAUCE

Snacking on a piece of fruit may not feel like something special. Yet somehow, a skewer of colorful fruit served with a dipping sauce feels like a real treat.

For optimum flavor, use seasonal fruit. Choose berries and melon in the warmer months or apples and bananas during cooler months. Supplement with year-round favorites like pineapple and grapes.

When using fruits that oxidize, like bananas, apples, or pears, brush their surface lightly with lemon juice after cutting to prevent discoloration.

SERVES 4 / PREP TIME: 15 MINUTES OR LESS / TOTAL TIME: 15 MINUTES OR LESS

---

3 cups berries or fresh fruit, cut into
  1-inch pieces
1 (6-ounce) container nonfat plain
  yogurt

1 tablespoon light brown sugar
1 tablespoon orange juice

Thread the fruits onto four 6-inch bamboo skewers, alternating types of fruit for better presentation.

    In a bowl, combine yogurt, sugar, and orange juice. Divide into four small cups and serve alongside fruit kebabs.

Per Serving	
Calories	80
Calories from Fat	0
Total Fat	0.0 g
Saturated Fat	0.1 g
Trans Fat	0.0 g
Polyunsaturated Fat	0.1 g
Monounsaturated Fat	0.0 g
Cholesterol	5 mg
Sodium	35 mg
Total Carbohydrate	18 g
Dietary Fiber	2 g
Sugars	15 g
Protein	3 g

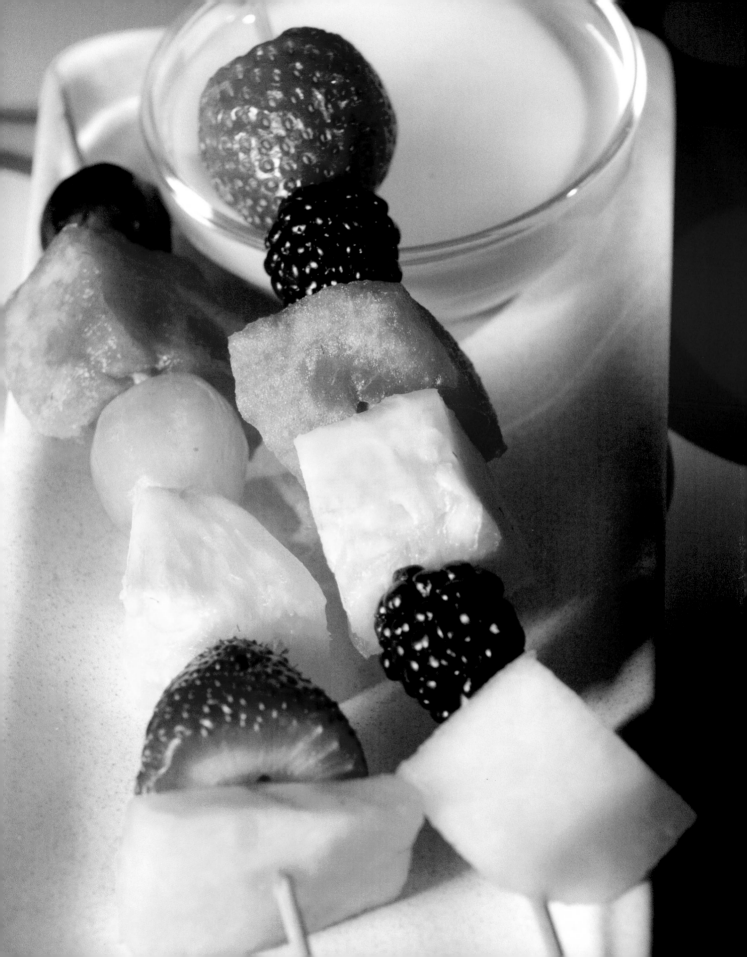

HOMEMADE BAKED TORTILLA CHIPS

These baked chips are a more healthful way to enjoy this treat.
Serve with Fresh Tomato Salsa or Tomatillo Salsa (pages 163 and 164).

Using a pizza cutter is an easy way to cut tortillas.

SERVES 4 / PREP TIME: 15 MINUTES OR LESS / TOTAL TIME: 15 MINUTES OR LESS

---

4 (6-inch) corn tortillas   Kosher or sea salt
1 teaspoon canola oil

Preheat the oven to 400 degrees. Lightly coat a baking sheet with nonstick cooking spray.

Using a pastry brush, dab tortillas with oil, or drizzle $1/4$ teaspoon oil on each tortilla and spread with a fingertip or the back of a spoon. Stack tortillas and cut into sixths. Arrange on the baking sheet and sprinkle lightly with salt.

Bake for 7 to 10 minutes, or until crisp.

Per Serving	
Calories	60
Calories from Fat	20
Total Fat	2.0 g
Saturated Fat	0.2 g
Trans Fat	0.0 g
Polyunsaturated Fat	0.7 g
Monounsaturated Fat	0.8 g
Cholesterol	0 mg
Sodium	10 mg
Total Carbohydrate	11 g
Dietary Fiber	2 g
Sugars	0 g
Protein	1 g

FRESH TOMATO SALSA

Salsa is not just for chips. A couple of spoonfuls over grilled chicken or fish transforms a simple main course into something memorable.

Adjust the salsa to taste, adding more onion, garlic, jalapeño, or hot sauce for pungency, or lime for tartness. Just be sure to start with ripe, flavorful tomatoes.

SERVES 8 / PREP TIME: 15 MINUTES OR LESS / TOTAL TIME: 15 MINUTES OR LESS

2 large ripe tomatoes, seeded and
 chopped
3 tablespoons chopped red onion
1 garlic clove, minced, or to taste
1 jalapeño, seeded and finely chopped

1/3 cup chopped fresh cilantro
1 tablespoon fresh lime juice, or
 to taste
Hot sauce, such as Tabasco
Salt and freshly ground black pepper

In a bowl, combine tomatoes, onion, garlic, jalapeño, and cilantro. Add lime juice and hot sauce and stir to combine. Season with salt and pepper. Taste and adjust seasonings as desired.

A jalapeño's heat can vary dramatically from pepper to pepper. Taste and adjust as needed. Use caution when chopping jalapeños to prevent their oils from touching your skin and eyes. Hold the tip with a piece of plastic wrap or use gloves to protect yourself.

Per Serving
Calories 15
 Calories from Fat 0
Total Fat . . . . 0.0 g
 Saturated Fat . . . . 0.0 g
 Trans Fat . . . . 0.0 g
 Polyunsaturated Fat . . . . 0.1 g
 Monounsaturated Fat . . . . . . 0.0 g
Cholesterol . . . . 0 mg
Sodium . . . . 0 mg
Total Carbohydrate . . . . 3 g
 Dietary Fiber . . . . 1 g
 Sugars . . . . 2 g
Protein . . . . 1 g

TOMATILLO SALSA

This salsa, which uses canned tomatillos and jalapeños for convenience, gets a burst of vibrancy from the addition of a healthy dose of fresh cilantro.

Serve salsa as a dip with chips, or use as it as a topping for grilled fish, chicken, or tacos.

SERVES 16 / PREP TIME: 15 MINUTES OR LESS / TOTAL TIME: 15 MINUTES OR LESS

1 small onion, quartered
1 (11-ounce can) tomatillos, drained

½ cup sliced canned nacho jalapeño slices
1 cup fresh cilantro

In a food professor, pulse onion two or three times. Add tomatillos, jalapeño slices with some juice, and cilantro and pulse until well combined.

Fresh tomatillos resemble green tomatoes but have a paper-like husk over the stem end. Used in many Latin American green sauces, tomatillos add tartness and texture.

Per Serving	
Calories	10
Calories from Fat	0
Total Fat	0.0 g
Saturated Fat	0.0 g
Trans Fat	0.0 g
Polyunsaturated Fat	0.1 g
Monounsaturated Fat	0.0 g
Cholesterol	0 mg
Sodium	105 mg
Total Carbohydrate	2 g
Dietary Fiber	0 g
Sugars	1 g
Protein	0 g

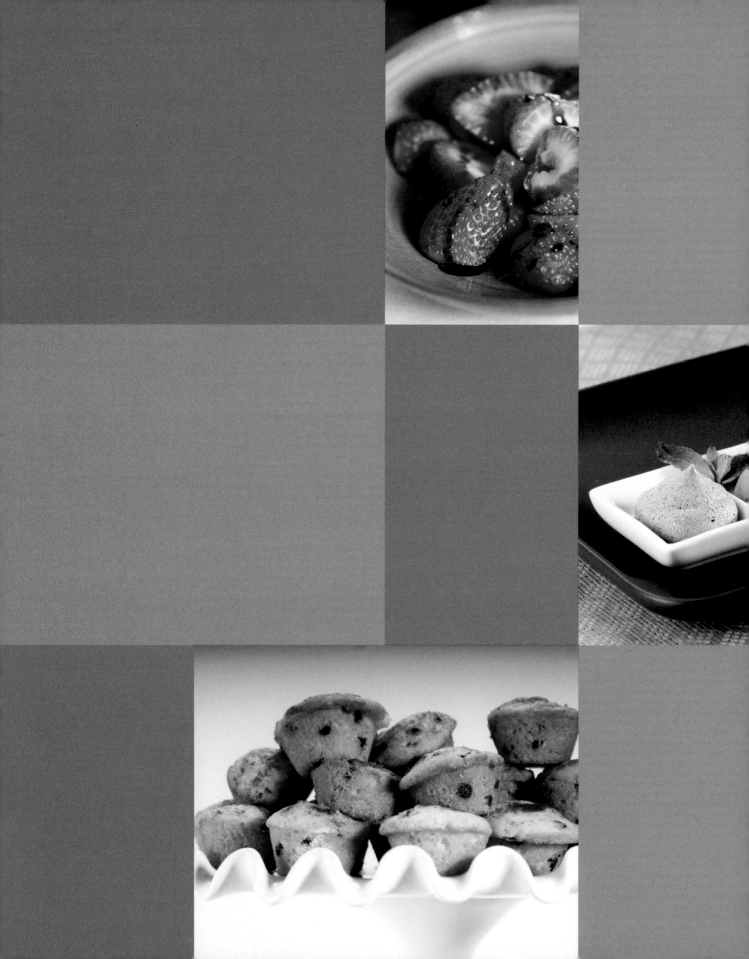

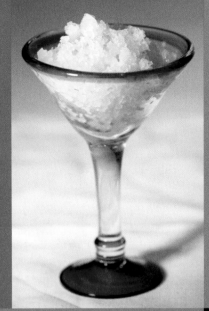

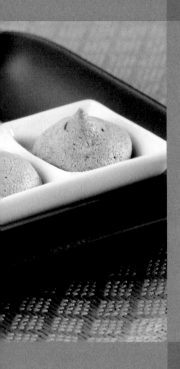

DESSERTS

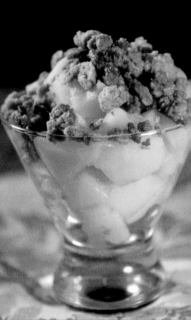

Who among us doesn't enjoy ending a meal with a sweet treat? A little slice of heaven can be good for the soul—without being bad for the waist. Indulge your sweet tooth in a small way, such as with our Two-Bite Brownies, or with a decadent-seeming fruit dessert, like the Microwave "Baked" Apples. This collection of truly delicious treats will have you leaving the table happy and satisfied.

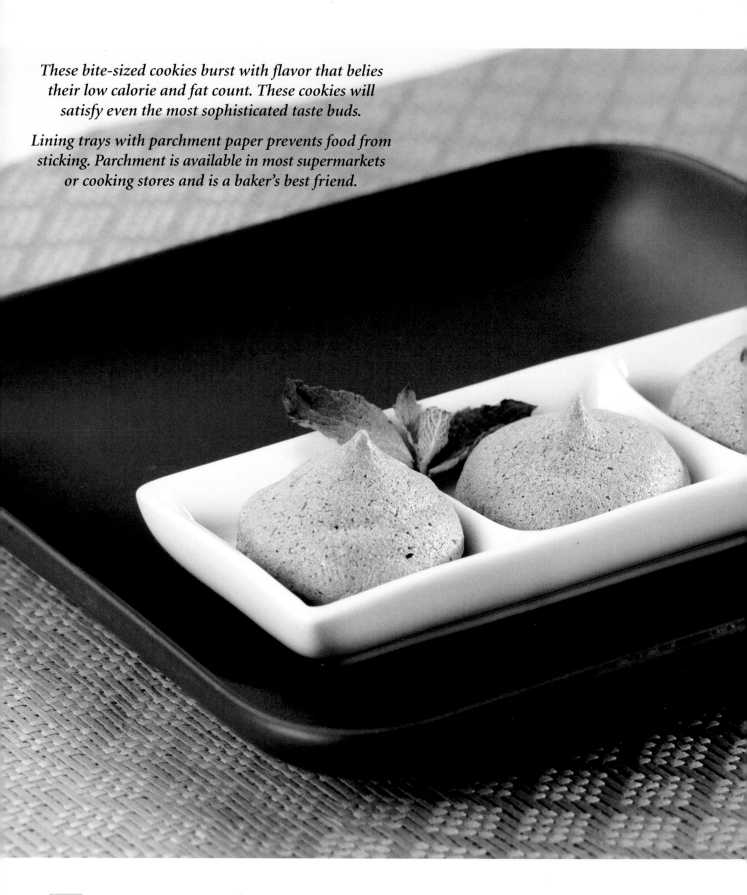

These bite-sized cookies burst with flavor that belies their low calorie and fat count. These cookies will satisfy even the most sophisticated taste buds.

Lining trays with parchment paper prevents food from sticking. Parchment is available in most supermarkets or cooking stores and is a baker's best friend.

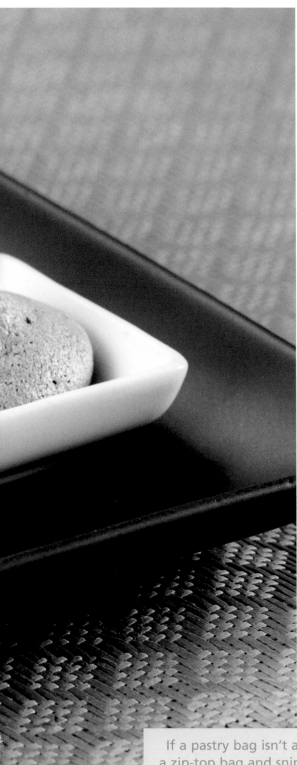

MINT-CHOCOLATE MERINGUE COOKIES

MAKES ABOUT 60 COOKIES / PREP TIME: 15 MINUTES OR LESS
TOTAL TIME: 45 MINUTES OR LESS

3 egg whites
$1/8$ teaspoon cream of tartar
$2/3$ cup granulated sugar
$1/4$ cup unsweetened cocoa powder, sifted
$1/4$ teaspoon mint extract
$1/3$ cup mini chocolate chips or finely chopped bittersweet
  chocolate

Preheat the oven to 300 degrees. Line two baking sheets with parchment paper, securing the edges with tape.

With an electric mixer, beat the egg whites and cream of tartar until soft peaks form. Gradually add sugar, 1 tablespoon at a time. Add cocoa powder and beat until the mixture becomes glossy. Add mint extract. Gently fold in chips.

Place mixture in a pastry bag fitted with a $1/2$- or $3/4$-inch tip. Pipe 1-inch rounds onto the parchment, leaving 1 to 2 inches between cookies. With damp fingertips, press down any peaks.

Bake for 25 to 30 minutes, rotating pans halfway through baking. Place baking sheets on a cooling rack for 10 minutes before peeling cookies off the parchment.

If a pastry bag isn't available, spoon mixture into a zip-top bag and snip a $1/2$-inch hole in the bottom corner of the bag. Batter can also be dropped with a tablespoon onto the parchment.

Per Serving	
Calories	15
Calories from Fat	0
Total Fat	0.0 g
Saturated Fat	0.2 g
Trans Fat	0.0 g
Polyunsaturated Fat	0.0 g
Monounsaturated Fat	0.1 g
Cholesterol	0 mg
Sodium	0 mg
Total Carbohydrate	3 g
Dietary Fiber	0 g
Sugars	3 g
Protein	0 g

ALMOND MACAROONS

When you want something sweet and satisfying, choose cookies that deliver intense flavor, like these macaroons. Almond paste, found in cans or tubes in the baking section of the grocery store, is the secret ingredient in these easy-to-make cookies.

Because these cookies have a tendency to stick, lining the baking sheets with parchment paper is highly recommended. Using insulated baking sheets or double stacking sheets also prevents the bottoms from overcooking.

These cookies can also be dropped by tablespoon, but using a piping bag speeds the prep time and guarantees perfect circles.

MAKES ABOUT 24 COOKIES / PREP TIME: 15 MINUTES OR LESS / TOTAL TIME: 45 MINUTES OR LESS

1 (7- or 8-ounce) package almond paste
1 cup confectioners sugar
2 tablespoons all-purpose flour

¼ teaspoon salt
2 egg whites

Preheat the oven to 350 degrees. Line two baking sheets, preferably the insulated variety, with parchment paper, securing the edges with tape.

In a food processor, pulse almond paste until powdery. Add confectioners sugar, flour, and salt and process until well blended and smooth. Add egg whites and process until blended and smooth.

Place mixture in a pastry bag fitted with a ½- or ¾-inch tip. Pipe 1-inch rounds onto the parchment, leaving 1 to 2 inches between cookies. With damp fingertips, press down any peaks.

Bake for 10 to 15 minutes, or until lightly golden. Place baking sheets on a cooling rack for 10 minutes before peeling cookies off the parchment.

If a pastry bag isn't available, spoon mixture into a zip-top bag and snip a ½-inch hole in the bottom corner of the bag. Batter can also be dropped with a tablespoon onto the parchment.

Per Serving	
Calories	60
Calories from Fat	20
Total Fat	2.5 g
Saturated Fat	0.2 g
Trans Fat	0.0 g
Polyunsaturated Fat	0.5 g
Monounsaturated Fat	1.5 g
Cholesterol	0 mg
Sodium	30 mg
Total Carbohydrate	9 g
Dietary Fiber	0 g
Sugars	8 g
Protein	1 g

TWO-BITE BROWNIES

There are no "bad" foods, just some that should be enjoyed in moderation. Just "two bites" of these intensely flavored brownies should satisfy any chocoholic's craving.

MAKES 20 TO 24 BROWNIES / PREP TIME: 15 MINUTES OR LESS / TOTAL TIME: 30 MINUTES OR LESS

½ cup all-purpose flour
¼ cup unsweetened cocoa powder
¼ teaspoon baking powder
Pinch salt
⅓ cup butter, melted

⅔ cup granulated sugar
1 teaspoon vanilla extract
1 egg, beaten
2 tablespoons mini chocolate chips, optional

Preheat the oven to 350 degrees. Lightly coat two mini-muffin tins with nonstick cooking spray.

In a bowl, combine flour, cocoa, baking powder, and salt.

In a bowl, combine butter, sugar, and vanilla. Add egg and beat until well blended. Add dry ingredients and stir well to combine. Stir in chocolate chips. Spoon heaping teaspoons into muffin cups.

Bake for 8 to 12 minutes, or until tops just bounce back when touched. Do not overbake. Leave in tins for 5 minutes before removing to a cooling rack.

Too tempting to have extra brownies around? No problem. Just pop extras in the freezer to enjoy later.

Per Serving
Calories 70
  Calories from Fat 30
Total Fat . . . . 3.5 g
  Saturated Fat . . . . 2.1 g
  Trans Fat . . . . 0.0 g
  Polyunsaturated Fat . . . . 0.2 g
  Monounsaturated Fat . . . . . . 0.9 g
Cholesterol . . . . 20 mg
Sodium . . . . 30 mg
Total Carbohydrate . . . . 10 g
  Dietary Fiber . . . . 0 g
  Sugars . . . . 7 g
Protein . . . . 1 g

"DECONSTRUCTED" APPLE CRISP

Instead of a typical crisp where everything is baked together,
this version combines all the elements of a crisp, but cooks them separately,
so each component retains its own structure. It also keeps sugar and fat to a minimum.

For an added treat, top with frozen or regular vanilla yogurt.

SERVES 4 / PREP TIME: 30 MINUTES OR LESS / TOTAL TIME: 45 MINUTES OR LESS

¼ cup all-purpose or whole wheat flour

2 tablespoons light brown sugar

2 tablespoons rolled oats

¼ teaspoon ground cinnamon

2 tablespoons cold butter, cut into
   ½-inch pieces

4 apples, peeled, cored, and cut into
   1-inch pieces

2 tablespoons fresh lemon juice

2 tablespoons granulated sugar

3 tablespoons water

Preheat the oven to 375 degrees. Line a baking sheet with parchment paper or lightly coat with nonstick cooking spray.

In a food processor, pulse flour, brown sugar, oats, and cinnamon to combine. Add butter and process until mixture is moistened throughout and dough begins to darken. Using the pulse button, process until moistened and pieces can be squeezed into small clumps.

On the baking sheet, spread ¼- to ¾-inch clumps to cover the sheet so there are different-sized pieces (it's ok to have some crumbs).

Bake for 4 to 5 minutes, toss clumps to redistribute, and bake for 5 to 7 minutes, or until crunchy and cooked through. Watch carefully during the last minutes of baking; the pieces should darken and harden but not overcook. You might need to stir more frequently for even cooking. Set aside to cool. The pieces will continue to firm up upon standing.

Meanwhile, in a saucepan over medium heat, combine apples, lemon juice, sugar, and water and stir to combine. Cook for 10 to 15 minutes, or until apples soften. Add additional water, 1 tablespoon at a time, if mixture begins to dry out or starts to stick to the pan. Set aside to cool.

Divide apples in individual bowls and top with crumbles.

Good apples for cooking include
Golden Delicious, Granny Smith, Jonathan,
McIntosh, and Gravenstein varieties.

Per Serving

Calories 210
   Calories from Fat 55
Total Fat . . . . 6.0 g
   Saturated Fat . . . . 3.7 g
   Trans Fat . . . . 0.0 g
   Polyunsaturated Fat . . . . 0.4 g
   Monounsaturated Fat . . . . . . 1.6 g
Cholesterol . . . . 15 mg
Sodium . . . . 45 mg
Total Carbohydrate . . . . 39 g
   Dietary Fiber . . . . 3 g
   Sugars . . . . 29 g
Protein . . . . 2 g

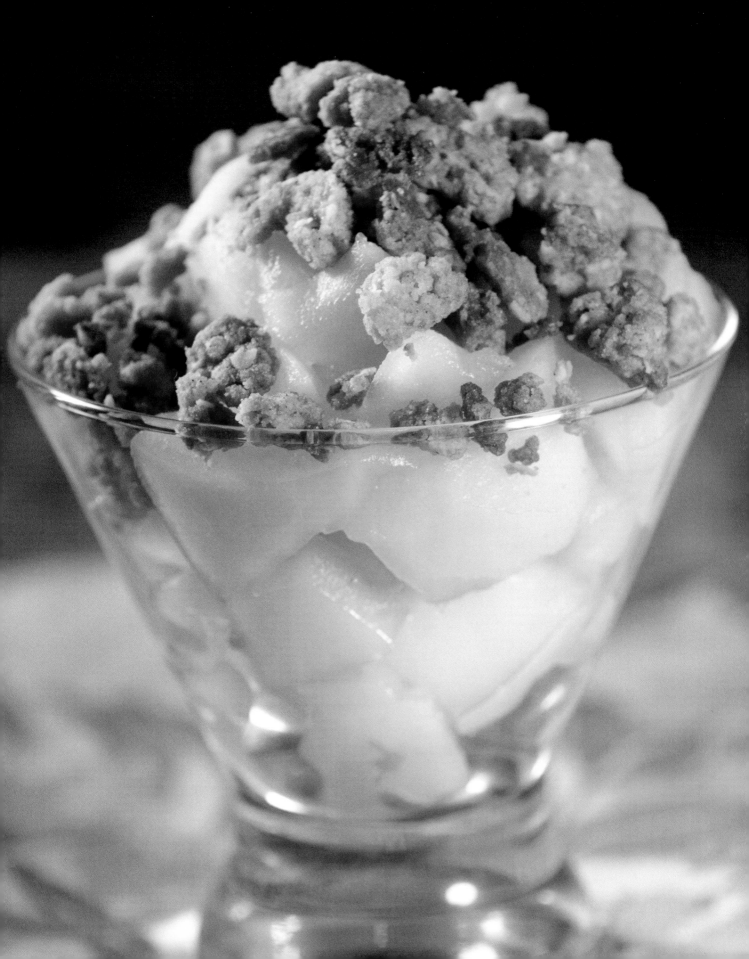

MOCK BERRY CRÈME BRÛLÉE

*There's no reason to deprive yourself of all things sweet just because
you are eating healthfully. This easy custard-like dessert of fresh berries
and sweetened yogurt is topped with a layer of brown sugar.
A quick trip under the broiler melts the sugar for a creamy, gooey,
fruity treat reminiscent of the not-so-good-for-you restaurant favorite.*

SERVES 1 / PREP TIME: 15 MINUTES OR LESS / TOTAL TIME: 15 MINUTES OR LESS

½ cup hulled and halved strawberries,
  raspberries, blueberries, or blackberries
3 tablespoons nonfat vanilla yogurt,
  divided

1 to 2 teaspoons light brown sugar

Position an oven rack 4 to 6 inches from the heat and preheat the broiler.

In a bowl, combine the berries and 2 tablespoons yogurt. Place in a 6-ounce ovenproof ramekin. Spread the remaining 1 tablespoon yogurt on top and sprinkle with enough brown sugar to coat the top in a thin, even layer.

Place the dish under the broiler and broil until the sugar melts, rotating the dish for even browning. The sugar can brown quickly, so pay attention to prevent burning.

Per Serving	
Calories	55
Calories from Fat	0
Total Fat	0.0 g
Saturated Fat	0.0 g
Trans Fat	0.0 g
Polyunsaturated Fat	0.1 g
Monounsaturated Fat	0.0 g
Cholesterol	0 mg
Sodium	25 mg
Total Carbohydrate	13 g
Dietary Fiber	2 g
Sugars	10 g
Protein	2 g

OATMEAL–RAISIN COOKIES

Unlike most recipes for oatmeal cookies, which call for white flour, granulated sugar, and a lot of fat, these are made with whole wheat flour, brown sugar, maple syrup, loads of oats, and only four tablespoons of butter.

MAKES ABOUT 26 COOKIES / PREP TIME: 15 MINUTES OR LESS / TOTAL TIME: 30 MINUTES OR LESS

1/4 cup butter, room temperature
1/4 cup light brown sugar
2 tablespoons maple syrup
1 egg
1/2 teaspoon vanilla

1/2 cup whole wheat flour
1/2 teaspoon baking soda
Pinch salt
1 cup rolled oats
1/2 cup raisins

Preheat the oven to 350 degrees. Line a baking sheet with parchment paper or lightly coat with nonstick cooking spray.

With an electric mixer, beat butter and sugar. Add syrup, egg, and vanilla and beat until well blended. Add flour, baking soda, and salt and beat until just combined. Scrape down sides, add oats and raisins, and beat to incorporate.

Drop the batter on the parchment by the tablespoon, leaving 1 to 2 inches between cookies.

Bake for 12 to 14 minutes, or until golden. Leave for 5 minutes before removing to a cooling rack.

Store cookies in an airtight container for optimum freshness.

Per Serving
Calories 60
    Calories from Fat 20
Total Fat . . . . 2.0 g
    Saturated Fat . . . . 1.2 g
    Trans Fat . . . . 0.0 g
    Polyunsaturated Fat . . . . 0.2 g
    Monounsaturated Fat . . . . . . 0.6 g
Cholesterol . . . . 15 mg
Sodium . . . . 40 mg
Total Carbohydrate . . . . 9 g
    Dietary Fiber . . . . 1 g
    Sugars . . . . 5 g
Protein . . . . 1 g

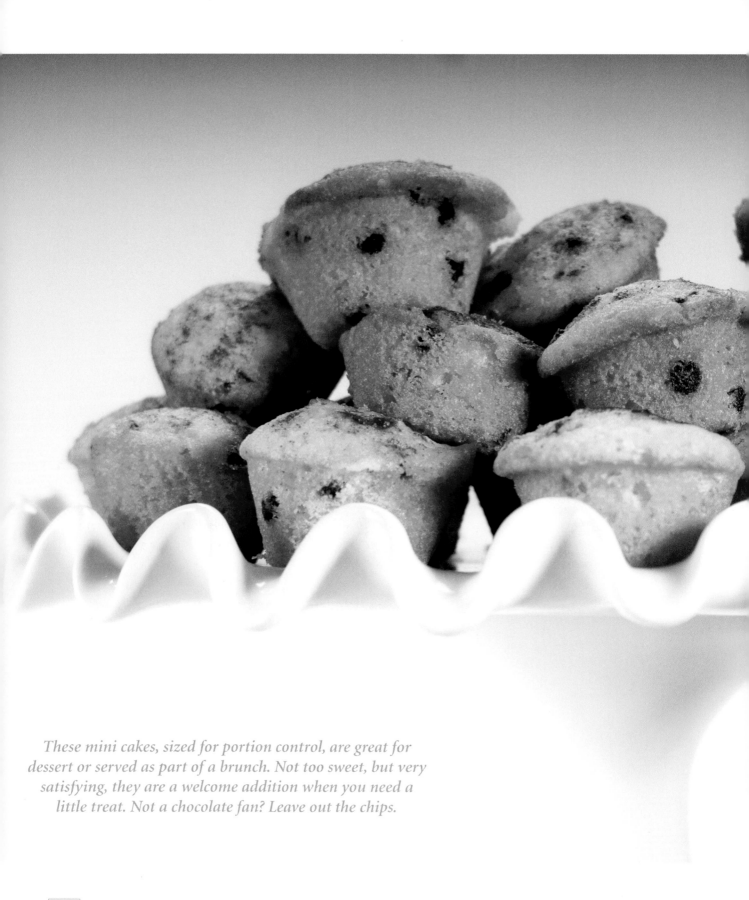

These mini cakes, sized for portion control, are great for dessert or served as part of a brunch. Not too sweet, but very satisfying, they are a welcome addition when you need a little treat. Not a chocolate fan? Leave out the chips.

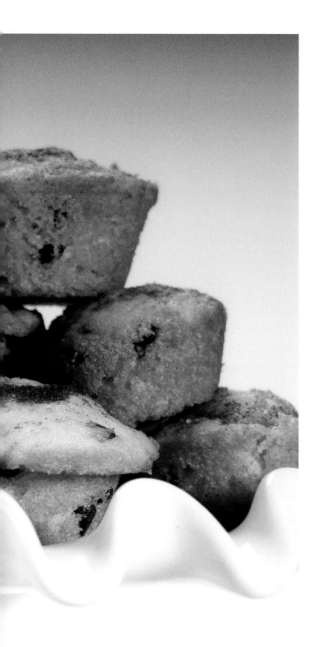

CHOCOLATE CHIP–SOUR CREAM COFFEE BABYCAKES

MAKES 24 CAKES / PREP TIME: 15 MINUTES OR LESS
TOTAL TIME: 30 MINUTES OR LESS

1/3 cup butter, room temperature
1/2 cup granulated sugar
1 egg
1/2 cup regular sour cream
1 teaspoon vanilla
1 cup all-purpose flour
3/4 teaspoon baking soda
1/4 cup mini chocolate chips
2 teaspoons cinnamon-sugar

Preheat the oven to 350 degrees. Lightly coat two mini-muffin tins with nonstick cooking spray.

With an electric mixer, beat butter and sugar. Add egg, sour cream, and vanilla and beat until well blended. Add flour and baking soda and beat until just combined. Scrape down sides and stir in chocolate chips. Spoon heaping teaspoons into muffin cups. Sprinkle with cinnamon-sugar.

Bake for 8 to 12 minutes, or until tops just bounce back when touched. Leave in tins for 5 minutes before removing to a cooling rack.

Make your own cinnamon-sugar by combining 1/4 cup granulated sugar with 1 tablespoon cinnamon. Store in an airtight container.

Per Serving	
Calories	80
Calories from Fat	35
Total Fat	4 g
Saturated Fat	2.6 g
Trans Fat	0.0 g
Polyunsaturated Fat	0.2 g
Monounsaturated Fat	1.1 g
Cholesterol	20 mg
Sodium	65 mg
Total Carbohydrate	10 g
Dietary Fiber	0 g
Sugars	6 g
Protein	1 g

MICROWAVE "BAKED" APPLES

*Using the microwave makes quick cooking of this classic "baked" dessert.
Use firm apples, like Granny Smith or Golden Delicious, which are good for baking,
and fill them with your favorite nuts and dried fruit.*

*In most microwaves, 6 minutes should be enough time for the apples
to release a bit of their juice and become tender. If your microwave
cooks quickly, check after 5 minutes.*

SERVES 4 / PREP TIME: 15 MINUTES OR LESS / TOTAL TIME: 15 MINUTES OR LESS

---

4 Granny Smith or Golden Delicious
  apples
1/4 cup chopped walnuts or pecans,
  toasted
1/4 cup dried and sweetened
  cranberries, such as Craisins

2 tablespoons light brown sugar
1/2 teaspoon ground cinnamon
1 tablespoon butter, quartered
2 tablespoons orange juice or apple
  juice

Cut out the stem and core of the apples, leaving a well. Do not cut all the way through the apple. (If you don't have an apple corer, use a paring knife to cut off the stem area and a grapefruit spoon to scoop out the remaining core and seeds.) Peel a strip of skin in a diagonal swirl.

In a bowl, combine nuts, cranberries, brown sugar, and cinnamon. Spoon mixture evenly into apples. Top with butter and press filling down inside apple.

Place apples in a microwave-safe 8-by-8-inch baking pan or casserole dish and drizzle with juice. Cover with plastic wrap.

Microwave on HIGH for 5 to 8 minutes, or until tender and some juices have been released. Carefully unwrap apples and spoon liquid over apples.

Per Serving	
Calories	200
Calories from Fat	70
Total Fat	8.0 g
Saturated Fat	2.3 g
Trans Fat	0.0 g
Polyunsaturated Fat	3.7 g
Monounsaturated Fat	1.4 g
Cholesterol	10 mg
Sodium	25 mg
Total Carbohydrate	34 g
Dietary Fiber	4 g
Sugars	27 g
Protein	2 g

CHOCOLATE–CHERRY FROZEN YOGURT

This fat-free icy dessert gives you the lingering impression of a dark chocolate–covered cherry.

SERVES 3 / PREP TIME: 15 MINUTES OR LESS / TOTAL TIME: 15 MINUTES OR LESS

2 cups frozen cherries
¼ cup nonfat vanilla yogurt
2 tablespoons chocolate syrup

In a food processor, combine cherries, yogurt, and chocolate syrup and process until smooth and creamy. Serve immediately.

Like many deeply colored fruits, cherries are full of powerful antioxidants called flavonoids.

Per Serving
Calories 175
  Calories from Fat 0
Total Fat . . . . 0.0 g
  Saturated Fat . . . . 0.1 g
  Trans Fat . . . . 0.0 g
  Polyunsaturated Fat . . . . 0.1 g
  Monounsaturated Fat . . . . . . 0.1 g
Cholesterol . . . . 0 mg
Sodium . . . . 20 mg
Total Carbohydrate . . . . 41 g
  Dietary Fiber . . . . 4 g
  Sugars . . . . 31 g
Protein . . . . 2 g

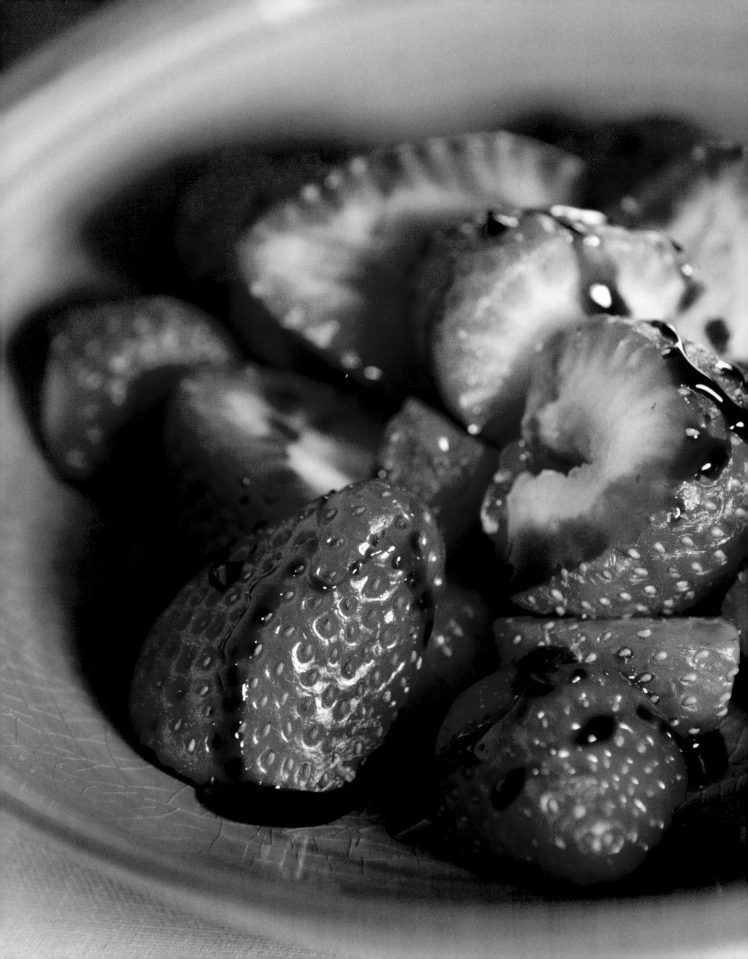

STRAWBERRIES WITH BALSAMIC GLAZE

This elegant dessert combination has become the darling of many fashionable restaurants. It's easily re-created at home at a fraction of the cost. While expensive aged balsamic vinegars are syrupy with a mild flavor, most balsamic vinegars are too acidic and thin to use as is in a dessert. Concentrating the syrup by boiling it until it thickens is a cheap but effective way to re-create the high-priced version. Adding a little sugar balances the flavors.

SERVES 4 / PREP TIME: 15 MINUTES OR LESS / TOTAL TIME: 30 MINUTES OR LESS

1 cup balsamic vinegar
2 tablespoons light brown sugar
2 cups sliced strawberries

In a heavy-bottomed saucepan over medium heat, combine vinegar and brown sugar. Cook for 10 to 20 minutes, or until thickened and syrupy, stirring occasionally. The mixture should reduce to between $1/3$ and $1/4$ cup. Set aside to cool. It will become thicker upon standing.

Divide strawberries in individual bowls and drizzle each serving with 1 teaspoon of glaze.

Per Serving
Calories 50
  Calories from Fat 0
Total Fat . . . . 0.0 g
  Saturated Fat . . . . 0.0 g
  Trans Fat . . . . 0.0 g
  Polyunsaturated Fat . . . . 0.1 g
  Monounsaturated Fat . . . . . . 0.0 g
Cholesterol . . . . 0 mg
Sodium . . . . 0 mg
Total Carbohydrate . . . . 13 g
  Dietary Fiber . . . . 2 g
  Sugars . . . . 9 g
Protein . . . . 1 g

ORANGE–CHERRY BISCOTTI

Biscotti, "twice baked" cookies, are crunchy delights.
They are wonderful served alongside coffee or an after-dinner drink.
Mix and match your favorite dried fruits or nuts.

MAKES 16 TO 18 BISCOTTI / PREP TIME: 15 MINUTES OR LESS / TOTAL TIME: 1 HOUR AND 15 MINUTES OR LESS

1 egg
1/2 cup granulated sugar
1/2 teaspoon vanilla extract
1 cup all-purpose flour
1/2 teaspoon baking powder

1/4 teaspoon baking soda
1/4 teaspoon salt
1/2 cup dried cherries
1/3 cup slivered almonds, toasted
Grated zest of 1 orange

Preheat the oven to 350 degrees. Line a baking sheet with parchment paper or lightly coat with nonstick cooking spray.

With an electric mixer, beat egg, sugar, and vanilla. On low speed, add flour, baking powder, baking soda, and salt. Initially, dough will be dry and crumbly. Continue mixing until dough begins to take form. Add cherries, almonds, and orange zest. Lightly coat a work surface with flour and scrape dough out onto surface. Lightly coat hands with flour and knead dough briefly until it is soft and not sticky (8 to 10 times). Shape dough into a log 8 to 10 inches long, 2 inches wide, and 1 inch high. Carefully place on the baking sheet.

Bake for 25 to 30 minutes or until well risen, lightly browned, and firm to the touch. Remove from the oven and reduce oven temperature to 325 degrees.

Cool log on the baking sheet for 5 to 10 minutes, or until warm but not too hot to handle. Transfer log to a cutting board. Using a serrated or sharp knife, cut diagonal 1/2-inch slices. Use a firm and fast cutting motion to prevent crumbling. Lay biscotti flat on the baking sheet. Bake for 10 minutes, flip biscotti over and bake for 5 to 10 minutes, or until golden, firm, and dry. Cookies might be slightly soft in center but will harden as they cool. Leave for 2 minutes before removing to a cooling rack.

Per Serving	
Calories	85
Calories from Fat	20
Total Fat	2.0 g
Saturated Fat	0.2 g
Trans Fat	0.0 g
Polyunsaturated Fat	0.4 g
Monounsaturated Fat	1.0 g
Cholesterol	15 mg
Sodium	75 mg
Total Carbohydrate	16 g
Dietary Fiber	1 g
Sugars	9 g
Protein	2 g

HOMEMADE BERRY FROZEN YOGURT

Creamy, gooey frozen yogurt is just a moment away with this food processor version.
It's the fastest way to get a healthful fresh-tasting dessert on the table.
Keep bags of fruit in the freezer for "dessert emergencies."

SERVES 6 / PREP TIME: 15 MINUTES OR LESS / TOTAL TIME: 15 MINUTES OR LESS

1 (16-ounce) package frozen strawberries or other berries
1 (6-ounce) container nonfat plain yogurt

⅓ cup plus 2 tablespoons confectioners sugar

Defrost the strawberries in the microwave on 30% power for 45 seconds to 1 minute. They should still feel frozen.

In a food processor, combine the berries, yogurt, and confectioners sugar and process until creamy and smooth. Serve immediately.

Per Serving	
Calories	75
Calories from Fat	0
Total Fat	0.0 g
Saturated Fat	0.0 g
Trans Fat	0.0 g
Polyunsaturated Fat	0.0 g
Monounsaturated Fat	0.0 g
Cholesterol	0 mg
Sodium	20 mg
Total Carbohydrate	18 g
Dietary Fiber	2 g
Sugars	14 g
Protein	2 g

PINK GRAPEFRUIT GRANITA

A granita—flavored shaved ice—is a light and refreshing way to end a meal. The citrusy zing of grapefruit makes it even more invigorating.

To get the right consistency, it's necessary to periodically scrape the mixture as it's freezing, to "slush" it up. Make sure you clear room in the freezer for the baking pan ahead of time! If your granita solidifies too much, pulse in a food processor just before serving.

SERVES 6 / PREP TIME: 30 MINUTES / TOTAL TIME: 4 HOURS OR LESS

½ cup granulated sugar
1 cup boiling water

3 cups strained, fresh pink grapefruit
juice (4 to 5 grapefruits)
Grated zest of 1 grapefruit

In a heatproof bowl, combine sugar and water. Stir until sugar dissolves. Let cool. Add grapefruit juice and zest and stir to combine.

Pour into a shallow 13-by-9-inch baking pan. The mixture should be no deeper than 1 inch. Freeze for 1 to 2 hours, or until the edges and bottom turn to ice. Using a fork, scrape the crystals and stir to distribute. Return to freezer and repeat every hour, or until the mixture is light-textured and icy.

Grapefruit contains fiber, vitamin C, lycopene, and other phytonutrients. The more red the grapefruit, the more lycopene it contains. For fresher and juicier fruit, choose heavy, firm grapefruits with smooth skins.

Per Serving
Calories 115
　Calories from Fat 0
Total Fat . . . . 0.0 g
　Saturated Fat . . . . 0.0 g
　Trans Fat . . . . 0.0 g
　Polyunsaturated Fat . . . . 0.0 g
　Monounsaturated Fat . . . . . . 0.0 g
Cholesterol . . . . 0 mg
Sodium . . . . 0 mg
Total Carbohydrate . . . . 28 g
　Dietary Fiber . . . . 0 g
　Sugars . . . . 28 g
Protein . . . . 1 g

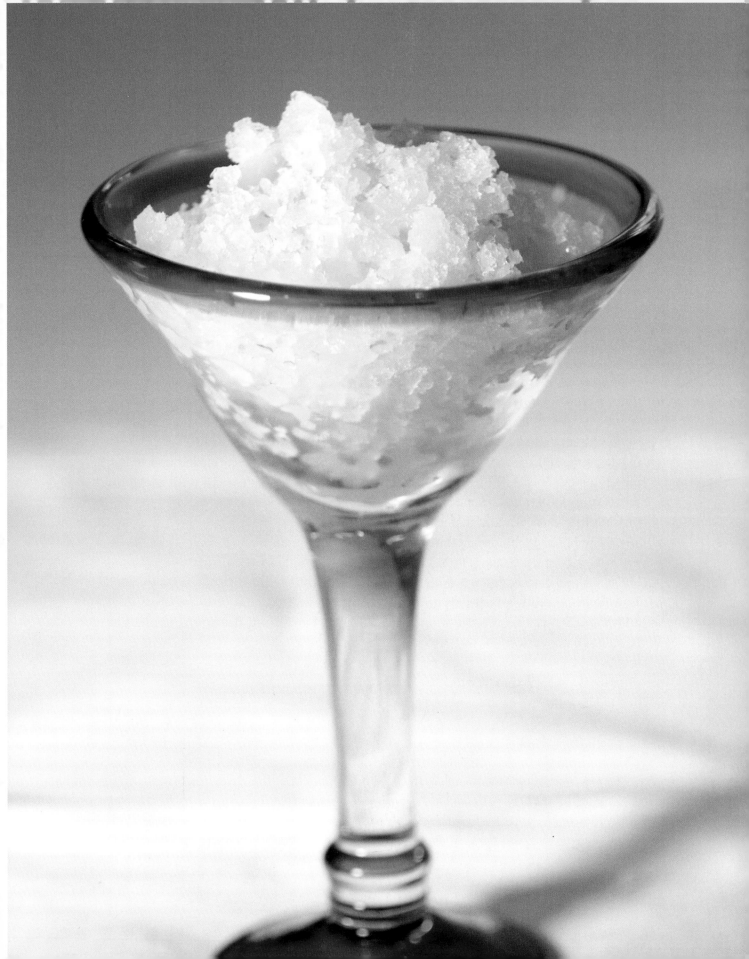

CHOCOLATE–ALMOND BISCOTTI

For those in need of a chocolate fix, try these biscotti.
They deliver rich flavor with satisfying crunch.

MAKES 16 TO 18 BISCOTTI / PREP TIME: 15 MINUTES OR LESS / TOTAL TIME: 1 HOUR AND 15 MINUTES OR LESS

---

1 egg
$1/2$ cup granulated sugar
$1/2$ teaspoon vanilla extract
1 cup all-purpose flour

3 tablespoons unsweetened cocoa
  powder
$1/2$ teaspoon baking soda
$1/4$ teaspoon salt
$1/3$ cup chopped almonds, toasted

Preheat the oven to 350 degrees. Line a baking sheet with parchment paper or lightly coat with nonstick cooking spray.

With an electric mixer, beat egg, sugar, and vanilla. On low speed, add flour, cocoa, baking soda, and salt. Initially, dough will be dry and crumbly. Continue mixing until dough begins to take form. Add almonds. Lightly coat a work surface with flour or cocoa and scrape dough out onto the surface. Lightly coat hands with flour and knead dough briefly until it is soft and not sticky (8 to 10 times). Shape dough into a log 8 to 10 inches long, 2 inches wide, and 1 inch high. Carefully place on the baking sheet.

Bake for 25 to 30 minutes or until well risen and firm to the touch. Remove from the oven and reduce oven temperature to 325 degrees.

Cool log on the baking sheet for 5 to 10 minutes, or until warm but not too hot to handle. Transfer log to a cutting board. Using a serrated or sharp knife, cut diagonal $1/2$-inch slices. Use a firm and fast cutting motion to prevent crumbling. Lay biscotti flat on the baking sheet. Bake for 10 minutes, flip biscotti over, and bake for 5 to 10 minutes, or until firm and dry. Cookies might be slightly soft in center but will harden as they cool. Leave for 2 minutes before removing to a cooling rack.

Per Serving	
Calories	70
Calories from Fat	15
Total Fat	1.5 g
Saturated Fat	0.3 g
Trans Fat	0.0 g
Polyunsaturated Fat	0.3 g
Monounsaturated Fat	0.9 g
Cholesterol	15 mg
Sodium	80 mg
Total Carbohydrate	13 g
Dietary Fiber	1 g
Sugars	7 g
Protein	2 g

CHOCOLATE-COVERED STRAWBERRIES

There's nothing like fruit dipped in chocolate to satisfy a sweet tooth. The sweetness of the berries is the perfect complement to the richness of the chocolate. It's the goods without the guilt.

This dessert is equally tasty with dried apricots or other dried fruits when strawberries are out of season.

SERVES 4 / PREP TIME: 15 MINUTES OR LESS / TOTAL TIME: 30 MINUTES OR LESS

4 squares German chocolate or 2 table-spoons semisweet chocolate chips

8 large strawberries

Place chocolate in a microwave-safe bowl and microwave on HIGH for 1 minute. Stir to combine. If necessary, heat for another 15 seconds.

Dip strawberries midway into melted chocolate and lay on wax paper to dry. Refrigerate for 10 to 20 minutes or until firm.

Per Serving	
Calories	40
Calories from Fat	20
Total Fat	2.0 g
Saturated Fat	1.0 g
Trans Fat	0.0 g
Polyunsaturated Fat	0.1 g
Monounsaturated Fat	0.7 g
Cholesterol	0 mg
Sodium	0 mg
Total Carbohydrate	7 g
Dietary Fiber	1 g
Sugars	5 g
Protein	0 g

HOW TO STOCK YOUR KITCHEN TO PROMOTE HEALTHY EATING

At the end of a long and busy day, the last thing you want to do is fight your way to the grocery store then rush home to put dinner on the table. Keeping healthy, flavorful ingredients on hand can help you put together a quick, easy, and satisfying meal in no time. Use these suggestions as a guide to make your own kitchen meal-ready on busy nights.

In Your Cupboard

☐ Whole grain cereals, rolled oats

☐ Beans: black, pinto, kidney, chickpeas, lentils, fat-free refried

☐ Rice: brown, long grain, basmati, Arborio, rice mixes

☐ Pasta: whole wheat spaghetti, fettuccine, penne, bowties, orzo, couscous

☐ Grains: kasha, quinoa, bulgur, cornmeal, whole wheat flour, bran, seasoned bread crumbs, panko, whole wheat bread, crackers

☐ Low-sodium canned vegetables: mixed vegetables, green beans, mushrooms, no-salt-added tomatoes (diced, whole, seasoned, sauce, paste)

☐ Canned fruits in juice: peaches, pineapple, pears, other favorites

☐ Dried fruits: cranberries, raisins, apricots, other favorites

☐ No-sugar-added applesauce

☐ Sun-dried tomatoes (not packed in oil)

☐ Sauces: pasta, pizza, salsa

☐ Soups: low-fat and reduced–sodium canned soups and stocks, bouillon and dried soup mixes

☐ Seafood and poultry: packaged tuna (in a can or pouch), salmon, minced clams, chicken

☐ Peanut butter (no-sugar-added or all-natural)

☐ Low-fat evaporated milk

☐ Capers

☐ Sauces and condiments: Worcestershire, soy, teriyaki, chili, hot pepper, ketchup, mustard (spicy, Dijon, honey), barbecue

☐ Vinegars: distilled white, cider, red wine, sherry, balsamic, rice wine

☐ Herbs and spices, salt and pepper

☐ Vanilla

☐ Oils: olive, canola, peanut, and nonfat cooking spray

☐ Onions, shallots, garlic

In Your Refrigerator

- ☐ Fresh vegetables and fruits
- ☐ 100% vegetable and fruit juices
- ☐ Nonfat or low-fat milk, buttermilk
- ☐ Nonfat or low-fat and no-sugar-added yogurt
- ☐ Cheeses (reduced-fat, where possible): cheddar, mozzarella, Swiss, Monterey Jack, Parmesan, cottage cheese, Neufchâtel (instead of cream cheese)
- ☐ Reduced–fat sour cream and mayonnaise
- ☐ Eggs and egg substitute
- ☐ Tofu
- ☐ Whole wheat and corn tortillas
- ☐ Salad dressings (reduced-fat or with olive oil)
- ☐ Minced garlic
- ☐ Olives
- ☐ Fresh herbs

In Your Freezer

- ☐ Frozen vegetables, fruits, and 100% juices
- ☐ Frozen chopped onion and chopped green pepper
- ☐ Breads: whole grain breads, dinner rolls, English muffins, bagels
- ☐ Poultry: skinless chicken breast, ground turkey breast, Cornish hens
- ☐ Seafood: tilapia, red snapper, salmon, orange roughy, cod, flounder, sole, shrimp, scallops
- ☐ Meats: extra-lean hamburger, lean cuts of beef (round, sirloin, flank steak, tenderloin), pork tenderloin

RECIPE MAKEOVERS 101: THREE STEPS TO HEALTHIER MEALS

If food doesn't taste good, it won't be eaten—it's as simple as that. Fortunately, there are many ways to cut down on the calories without sacrificing flavor. It's also easy to add extra nutrients by adding more fruits, vegetables, and whole grains. The recipes in this book follow these guidelines. Use the tips below to achieve the same great taste—with a lot fewer calories—in your own daily eating.

Step 1: Increase the vegetables, fruits, and whole grains each day.
Add fresh or dried fruits like banana slices, blueberries, or raisins to your cereal.

Add fresh or dried fruits like chopped apples, raisins, prunes, kiwi, or orange sections to green leafy salads.

Add dried fruits or vegetables to grain-based dishes, like rice or couscous.

Add chopped carrots, broccoli, or a mix of your favorite vegetables to soups, salads, and casseroles.

Add canned beans to soups, stews, and salads.

Substitute whole wheat flour for up to half (or more) of the white flour called for in a recipe.

Add ¹/₂ cup bran or quick-cooking oatmeal to meat loaf or casseroles.

Make muffins using oatmeal, bran, or whole wheat flour.

Use whole cornmeal when making cornbread.

Step 2: Lower the amount of calories.
The best ways to reduce calories in the dishes you make are to look for ways to cut down on fat and sugar. Try these tips:

In baked goods, reduce the fat by half (if a recipe calls for 1 cup of oil, use ¹/₂ cup). You can also reduce the sugar by half.

If making quick breads like banana, zucchini, or other sweet breads, cut the oil in half and replace with an equal amount of applesauce, mashed banana, or even canned pumpkin.

If a recipe calls for nuts, use half the amount but toast the nuts—this intensifies the flavor and saves on calories.

In egg-based dishes, replace half the eggs with egg whites, using two egg whites per egg. (If a recipe calls for two eggs, use one egg and two egg whites.)

Use evaporated (skim or whole) milk instead of cream in baked goods, sauces, and soups.

Use a puree of cooked potatoes, onion, and celery as a creamy base for soups instead of cream or half-and-half.

Use reduced-fat cheese when possible: low-fat cottage cheese, Neufchâtel (instead of cream cheese), part-skim mozzarella, and reduced-fat sharp cheddar.

Step 3: Cut back on high-fat meats.
Use leaner cuts of meat: look for the words "loin" or "round" in the name.

Use ground turkey breast in place of ground beef.

Trim all visible fat before cooking.

Cook poultry with the skin on to keep it moist, but remove skin before eating to reduce the fat content.

AMERICAN CANCER SOCIETY GUIDELINES ON NUTRITION AND PHYSICAL ACTIVITY

*Want to reduce your risk of cancer, heart disease, and diabetes?
If you are a nonsmoker, watching your weight, living a physically active lifestyle,
and eating well are the most important ways to improve your health and reduce
your risk of all these chronic diseases. The following nutrition and physical activity
recommendations offer the best advice available to reduce your risk of cancer:*

Maintain a healthy weight throughout life.
Balance caloric intake with physical activity.

Avoid excessive weight gain over the course of your life.

Achieve and maintain a healthy weight if currently overweight or obese.

Adopt a physically active lifestyle.
Adults should be moderately to vigorously active for at least 30 minutes, in addition to your usual activities, on 5 or more days of the week. Forty-five to 60 minutes of intentional physical activity are preferable.

Children and adolescents should engage in at least 60 minutes per day of moderate to vigorous physical activity at least 5 days per week.

Consume a healthy diet, with an emphasis on plant sources.
Choose foods and beverages in amounts that help achieve and maintain a healthy weight.

Eat five or more servings of a variety of vegetables and fruits each day.

Choose whole grains in preference to processed (refined) grains.

Limit consumption of processed and red meats.

If you drink alcoholic beverages, limit consumption.
Drink no more than one alcoholic drink per day for women or two per day for men.

INDEX

A

Almond(s)
Almond Macaroons, 170
Chocolate–Almond Biscotti, 186
paste, 170
Wheat Berry Salad with Almonds and Dried Cherries, 98
American Cancer Society guidelines on nutrition and physical activity, 191
Andouille sausage, 9
Apple cider
Whipped Cider Sweet Potatoes, 113
Apple(s)
Aromatic Butternut Squash and Apple Soup, 65
Braised Red Cabbage and Apples, 116
Carrot–Raisin–Apple Salad, 103
"Deconstructed" Apple Crisp, 172
Golden Delicious, 172, 178
Granny Smith, 172, 178
Gravenstein, 172
Jonathan, 172
McIntosh, 172
Microwave "Baked" Apples, 178
in *Pork Tenderloin Topped with Fall Fruits*, 31
Applesauce
Carrot–Applesauce Muffins, 142
Apricot(s)
Apricot–Orange Baked Chicken, 27
in *Dried Fruit Compote*, 145
nutrients in, 145
Arborio rice
in *Fig, Ginger, and Butternut Squash Risotto*, 52
in *Shrimp and Asparagus Risotto*, 11
Aromatic Butternut Squash and Apple Soup, 65
Arugula
Arugula and Parmigiano–Reggiano Salad, 109
Beet, Orange, and Arugula Salad, 96
Asian Beef Salad, 83
Asparagus
Lemon-Roasted Asparagus, 120

nutrients in, 120
Shrimp and Asparagus Risotto, 11
Avocado(s)
Crab Salad with Grapefruit, Avocado, and Baby Greens, 76
nutrients in, 91
Shrimp, Watermelon, and Avocado Salad, 91
storage, 91

B

Baked Eggs Florentine, 140
Balsamic vinegar
in *Strawberries with Balsamic Glaze*, 181
white, 102
Banana(s)
Banana Pancakes, 141
Strawberry–Banana Smoothie, 135
Barbecue Chicken Quesadilla, 75
Barley
about, 33
Chicken and Barley Stew, 33
Mushroom–Barley Soup, 71
Basil. *See also* Herb(s)
Tomato and Basil Frittata, 139
Basmati rice
about, 119
Basmati Rice and Chickpea Pilaf, 119
Beans. *See also* Black beans; Green beans
canned, 32
cannellini, 48, 67, 85
Chicken and White Bean Soup, 69
Great Northern, 69
green, 24, 57, 67, 117
kidney, 88
navy, 32, 67
pinto, 94
Quesadilla with Beans, Corn, and Green Chiles, 94
Ratatouille with Beans, 49
Shrimp, Bean, and Feta Bake, 48
Southwestern Bean Burgers, 88
Tuna–Bean Salad, 85
white kidney beans, 48

Beef
Asian Beef Salad, 83
lean ground, choosing, 46
in *Mini Meatloaves*, 46
in *Olé Pasta Casserole*, 22
Roast Beef Roll-Up, 97
Beet(s)
Beet, Orange, and Arugula Salad, 96
nutrients in, 96
Bell peppers. *See* Peppers
Beta-carotene, 37, 40, 106, 136, 145
Biscotti
Chocolate–Almond Biscotti, 186
Orange–Cherry Biscotti, 182
Black beans
Black Bean and Butternut Squash Chili, 43
Black Bean and Corn Salad, 115
Black Bean Soup with Cilantro Cream, 66
Blackberry(ies)
in *Mock Berry Crème Brûlée*, 174
Blueberry(ies)
Blueberry–Peach–Pomegranate Smoothie, 149
in *Brown Sugar Yogurt Parfait*, 131
in *Mock Berry Crème Brûlée*, 174
Braised Red Cabbage and Apples, 116
Bran
Buttermilk Bran Muffins, 137
Broccoli
Broccoli, Garlic, and Lemon Penne, 3
Chicken and Broccoli Stir-Fry, 37
Brown rice
Brown Rice Pilaf, 118
Portobellos Stuffed with Spinach, Brown Rice, and Feta, 21
in *Tomato–Fennel Tofu Bake*, 18
Brown Sugar Yogurt Parfait, 131
Brussels sprouts
about, 126
Roasted Brussels Sprouts, 126
Buckwheat noodles
in *Spicy Soba Salad*, 80
Bulgur
about, 111
in *Tabbouleh Salad*, 111

Burgers. *See also* Sandwiches
  Lamb Burgers with Tomato–Olive Relish, 89
  Southwestern Bean Burgers, 88
  Turkey Burgers with Cranberry Chutney, 86
  Wasabi Salmon Burgers, 5
Buttermilk
  Buttermilk Bran Muffins, 137
  in *Garlic Mashed Potatoes,* 108
Butternut squash
  Aromatic Butternut Squash and Apple Soup, 65
  Black Bean and Butternut Squash Chili, 43
  Fig, Ginger, and Butternut Squash Risotto, 52
B vitamins, 33, 50, 71

C

Cabbage
  Braised Red Cabbage and Apples, 116
  in *Caraway Cole Slaw,* 107
Calcium, 3
Calories, reducing, 190
Cannellini beans. *See* Beans
Canola oil
  nutrients in, 28, 32
Capers
  about, 159
Caraway Cole Slaw, 107
Carrot(s)
  Carrot–Applesauce Muffins, 142
  Carrot–Raisin–Apple Salad, 103
  Orange–Glazed Baby Carrots, 122
  Roasted Potatoes and Baby Carrots, 124
  vitamin A in, 103
Casseroles
  Olé Pasta Casserole, 22
  Tomato–Fennel Tofu Bake, 18
Celery
  nutrients in, 70
  storage, 70
Cheese. *See also* Feta cheese; Pizza;
  Quesadillas

  Arugula and Parmigiano–Reggiano Salad, 109
  Cheesy Pita Crisps, 152
  grating, 3
  Lower-Fat Mac-n-Cheese, 26
  reduced-fat, 26
Cherry(ies)
  Chocolate–Cherry Frozen Yogurt, 179
  Orange–Cherry Biscotti, 182
  Wheat Berry Salad with Almonds and Dried Cherries, 98
Chicken
  Apricot–Orange Baked Chicken, 27
  Barbecue Chicken Quesadilla, 75
  Chicken and Barley Stew, 33
  Chicken and Broccoli Stir-Fry, 37
  Chicken and White Bean Soup, 69
  Chicken Chili, 32
  Crunchy "Oven-Fried" Chicken Nuggets, 28
  Curried Chicken Salad, 79
  Greek Chicken and Tzatziki Pitas, 87
  Grilled Chicken Breasts with Pineapple Salsa, 4
  Grilled Teriyaki Chicken Kebabs, 38
  Mediterranean Chicken Salad, 81
  Moo Shu Chicken Lettuce Wraps, 55
  Moroccan Spiced Chicken with Vegetable Couscous, 42
  Quick Chicken Cacciatore, 39
  removing skin of, 27
  rotisserie, uses for, 69
  sausage, 8, 9
  Southwest Chicken Tortilla Soup, 64
  Stuffed Greek Chicken Breasts, 58
  Tandoori-Style Chicken, 19
Chicken broth, freezing, 33
Chickpea(s)
  Basmati Rice and Chickpea Pilaf, 119
  in *Moroccan Spiced Chicken with Vegetable Couscous,* 42
  in *Ratatouille with Beans,* 49
  in *Spinach, Portobello, and Roasted Red Pepper Salad,* 95
Chili
  Black Bean and Butternut Squash Chili, 43

  Chicken Chili, 32
Chili paste, 83
Chili-Spiced Popcorn, 156
Chocolate
  Chocolate–Almond Biscotti, 186
  Chocolate–Cherry Frozen Yogurt, 179
  Chocolate Chip–Sour Cream Coffee Babycakes, 177
  Chocolate-Covered Strawberries, 187
  Mint-Chocolate Meringue Cookies, 169
  Two-Bite Brownies, 171
Chunky Vegetable Salad, 102
Cilantro. *See also* Herb(s)
  Black Bean Soup with Cilantro Cream, 66
Cinnamon-sugar, 177
Clam(s)
  Red Clam Chowder, 70
  in *Seafood Stew,* 60
Coconut milk, 24
Cod
  in *Grilled Baja–Style Fish Tacos,* 13
  in *Provençal Fish,* 6
  in *Seafood Stew,* 60
Cole slaw
  Caraway Cole Slaw, 107
Cookie(s)
  Almond Macaroons, 169
  Chocolate–Almond Biscotti, 186
  Mint-Chocolate Meringue Cookies, 169
  Oatmeal–Raisin Cookies, 175
  Orange–Cherry Biscotti, 182
  piping with zip-top bag, 169, 170
  Two-Bite Brownies, 171
Corn
  Black Bean and Corn Salad, 115
  Quesadilla with Beans, Corn, and Green Chiles, 94
  Quinoa and Corn Salad with Rosemary, 93
  tortillas, fiber in, 23
Crab Salad with Grapefruit, Avocado, and Baby Greens, 76
Cranberry(ies)
  Ginger–Cranberry Granola, 148
  nutrients in, 86

Turkey Burgers with Cranberry Chutney, 86
Creamy Peanut Butter Dip, 158
Crunchy "Oven-Fried" Chicken Nuggets, 28
Curry
    Curried Chicken Salad, 79
    Green Curry Shrimp, 24
    Microwave Thai Red Curry Salmon, 14
Curry paste
    green, 24
    Thai red, 14

D

"Deconstructed" Apple Crisp, 172
Dried Fruit Compote, 145
Drinks
    Blueberry–Peach–Pomegranate Smoothie,
      149
    Raspberry–Peach Yogurt Smoothie, 132
    Strawberry–Banana Smoothie, 135
Dry foods to keep on hand, 188

E

Eggplant Spread, 123
Eggs
    Baked Eggs Florentine, 140
    Eggs-Traordinary Taco, 78
    Ham and Vegetable Frittata, 130
    Tomato and Basil Frittata, 139

F

Fennel
    Mussels with Fennel, Leek, and Grape
      Tomatoes, 16
    Tomato–Fennel Tofu Bake, 18
Feta cheese
    Portobellos Stuffed with Spinach, Brown
      Rice, and Feta, 21
    Shrimp, Bean, and Feta Bake, 48
    in *Stuffed Greek Chicken Breasts*, 58
Fettuccine. *See* Pasta
Fettuccine with Tomato–Herb Sauce, 56
Fiber, 3, 32, 33, 36, 37, 42, 48, 49, 71, 98,
    103, 106, 111, 124, 144, 145, 184
Fig, Ginger, and Butternut Squash Risotto, 52
Fish. *See* Seafood
Folate (folic acid), 3, 48, 56, 57, 71, 96, 120
Fresh Tomato Salsa, 163
Frittatas
    Ham and Vegetable Frittata, 130

Tomato and Basil Frittata, 139
Frozen desserts
    Chocolate–Cherry Frozen Yogurt, 179
    Homemade Berry Frozen Yogurt, 183
    Pink Grapefruit Granita, 184
Frozen foods to keep on hand, 190
Fruit. *See also* specific fruits
    dried, 52
    Dried Fruit Compote, 145
    frozen, 132
    Fruit Skewers with Yogurt Dipping
      Sauce, 160
    Fruity Morning Oatmeal, 144

G

Garlic Mashed Potatoes, 108
Ginger
    Fig, Ginger, and Butternut Squash Risotto,
      52
    Ginger–Cranberry Granola, 148
    Ginger-Poached Salmon with Orange and
      Honey, 15
    health benefits of, 15
    Whole Grain Gingerbread Waffles, 134
Golden Delicious apples. *See* Apples
Granny Smith apples. *See* Apples
Granola
    Ginger–Cranberry Granola, 148
    in *Brown Sugar Yogurt Parfait*, 131
Grapefruit
    Crab Salad with Grapefruit, Avocado, and
      Baby Greens, 76
    nutrients in, 76, 184
    Pink Grapefruit Granita, 184
    sectioning, 76
    selecting, 184
Great Northern beans. *See* Beans
Greek Chicken and Tzatziki Pitas, 87
Green beans
    Sautéed Green Beans and Grape Tomatoes,
      117
    Stir-Fried Pork, Green Beans, and Shiitake
      Mushrooms, 57
Green Curry Shrimp, 24
Greens and Herb Salad, 112
Grilled Baja–Style Fish Tacos, 13
Grilled Chicken Breasts with Pineapple
    Salsa, 4
Grilled Teriyaki Chicken Kebabs, 38

Grilled (foods)
    Asian Beef Salad, 83
    Grilled Baja–Style Fish Tacos, 13
    Grilled Chicken Breasts with Pineapple
      Salsa, 4
    Grilled Teriyaki Chicken Kebabs, 38

H

Halibut
    in *Grilled Baja–Style Fish Tacos*, 13
    in *Provençal Fish*, 6
Ham and Vegetable Frittata, 130
Herb(s). *See also* specific herbs
    Fettuccine with Tomato–Herb Sauce, 56
    Greens and Herb Salad, 112
    Oven-Roasted Herbed Turkey Breast, 7
    storing fresh, 112
    substituting fresh for dried, 39
Homemade Baked Tortilla Chips, 162
Homemade Berry Frozen Yogurt, 183
Homemade Pizza, 35
Honey
    Ginger-Poached Salmon with Orange and
      Honey, 15

I

Iron, 3, 16, 72, 93, 96, 103, 120, 144

J

Jalapeños
    handling, 163

K

Kidney beans. *See* Beans
Kitchen, stocking one's, 188–189

L

Lamb Burgers with Tomato–Olive Relish,
    89
Leek(s)
    Mussels with Fennel, Leek, and Grape
      Tomatoes, 16
    Savory Salmon and Leek Packets, 47
Lemon(s)
    Broccoli, Garlic, and Lemon Penne, 3
    Lemon-Roasted Asparagus, 120
Lentil(s)
    Lentil–Vegetable Soup, 72
    nutrients in, 72

Lower-Fat Mac-n-Cheese, 26
Lycopene, 6, 35, 49, 76, 184

M

Macaroni
  Lower-Fat Mac-n-Cheese, 26
Magnesium, 3, 48, 93, 144
Makeovers, recipe, 190
Mango(es)
  cutting tips, 40
  nutrients in, 40
  Poached Salmon with Mango Salsa,
    40
Mayonnaise
  horseradish, 97
  wasabi, 5
Mediterranean Chicken Salad, 81
Mediterranean Tuna Pâté, 159
Mexican "Lasagna," 53
Microwave "Baked" Apples, 178
Microwave cooking
  Microwave "Baked" Apples, 178
  Microwave Thai Red Curry Salmon, 14
  Pepperoni Tortilla Pizza, 155
  Veggie Tortilla Pizza, 157
Microwave Thai Red Curry Salmon, 14
Mini Meatloaves, 46
Mint-Chocolate Meringue Cookies, 169
Mock Berry Crème Brûlée, 174
Moo Shu Chicken Lettuce Wraps, 55
Moroccan Spiced Chicken with Vegetable
  Couscous, 42
Muffins
  Buttermilk Bran Muffins, 137
  Carrot–Applesauce Muffins, 142
Mushroom(s)
  Mushroom–Barley Soup, 71
  Portobellos Stuffed with Spinach, Brown
    Rice, and Feta, 21
  Spinach, Portobello, and Roasted Red
    Pepper Salad, 95
  Stir-Fried Pork, Green Beans, and Shiitake
    Mushrooms, 57
Mussels
  Mussels with Fennel, Leek, and Grape
    Tomatoes, 16
  nutrients in, 16
  in *Seafood Stew*, 60

N

Navy beans. *See* Beans
Nutrition guidelines, 191
Nuts
  storage, 148
  toasting, 21, 93

O

Oat(s)
  Fruity Morning Oatmeal, 144
  in *Ginger–Cranberry Granola*, 148
  nutrients in, 144
  Oatmeal–Raisin Cookies, 175
  Oatmeal–Raisin Scones, 147
Olé Pasta Casserole, 22
Olive oil
  extra-virgin, 56, 81
  nutrients in, 28, 56
Omega-3 fatty acids, 50
Orange(s)
  Apricot–Orange Baked Chicken, 27
  Beet, Orange, and Arugula Salad, 96
  Ginger-Poached Salmon with Orange and
    Honey, 15
  Orange–Cherry Biscotti, 182
  Orange–Glazed Baby Carrots, 122
Oven–Baked Potato Chips, 104
Oven-Roasted Herbed Turkey Breast, 7

P

Pancakes
  Banana Pancakes, 141
  Pumpkin-Spice Pancakes, 136
Panko, 5
Pantry supplies, 188
Parmigiano–Reggiano cheese
  Arugula and Parmigiano–Reggiano Salad,
    109
Parsley. *See also* Herb(s)
  nutrients in, 56
Pasta
  Broccoli, Garlic, and Lemon Penne, 3
  Fettuccine with Tomato–Herb Sauce,
    56
  Lower-Fat Mac-n-Cheese, 26
  Olé Pasta Casserole, 22
  in *Super Veggie Soup*, 67
  Whole Wheat Penne with Roasted
    Vegetable Sauce, 36

Peach(es)
  Blueberry–Peach–Pomegranate Smoothie,
    149
  Raspberry–Peach Yogurt Smoothie, 132
Peanut butter
  all-natural, 158
  Creamy Peanut Butter Dip, 158
  Tofu Stir-Fry with Peanut Sauce, 10
Pear(s)
  in *Pork Tenderloin Topped with Fall*
    Fruits, 31
Penne. *See* Pasta
Pepperoni Tortilla Pizza, 155
Peppers
  red and yellow, beta-carotene in, 37
  red, nutrients in, 57
  roasting, 95
  Spinach, Portobello, and Roasted Red
    Pepper Salad, 95
Pesto
  Steamed Pesto-Rolled Tilapia with
    Vegetables, 29
Physical activity guidelines, 191
Pineapple(s)
  Grilled Chicken Breasts with Pineapple
    Salsa, 4
Pine nuts
  toasting, 21, 93
Pink Grapefruit Granita, 184
Pinto beans. *See* Beans
Pita(s)
  Cheesy Pita Crisps, 152
  Greek Chicken and Tzatziki Pitas, 87
Pizza
  Homemade Pizza, 35
  Pepperoni Tortilla Pizza, 155
  Veggie Tortilla Pizza, 157
Poached (foods)
  Ginger-Poached Salmon with Orange and
    Honey, 15
  Poached Salmon with Mango Salsa, 40
Pomegranate juice
  Blueberry–Peach–Pomegranate Smoothie,
    149
Popcorn
  Chili-Spiced Popcorn, 156
  Rosemary Popcorn, 153
Pork
  Ham and Vegetable Frittata, 130

Pork Tenderloin Topped with Fall Fruits, 31
Stir-Fried Pork, Green Beans, and Shiitake
   Mushrooms, 57
Portobello(s)
   Portobellos Stuffed with Spinach, Brown
      Rice, and Feta, 21
   Spinach, Portobello, and Roasted Red
      Pepper Salad, 95
Potassium, 33, 37, 49, 70, 71, 72, 103, 108,
   145
Potato(es)
   Garlic Mashed Potatoes, 108
   Oven–Baked Potato Chips, 104
   Roasted Potatoes and Baby Carrots, 124
   Sweet Potato Fries, 106
   Whipped Cider Sweet Potatoes, 113
Protein, 10, 33, 50, 71, 72, 93, 98
Provençal Fish, 6
Prunes
   in Dried Fruit Compote, 145
   nutrients in, 145
Pumpkin
   nutrients in, 136
   Pumpkin-Spice Pancakes, 136

Q

Quesadillas
   Barbecue Chicken Quesadilla, 75
   Quesadilla with Beans, Corn, and Green
      Chiles, 94
Quick Chicken Cacciatore, 39
Quinoa
   about, 93
   nutrients in, 93
   Quinoa and Corn Salad with Rosemary, 93

R

Raisin(s)
   Carrot–Raisin–Apple Salad, 103
   Oatmeal–Raisin Cookies, 175
   Oatmeal–Raisin Scones, 147
Raspberry(ies)
   in Mock Berry Crème Brûlée, 174
   Raspberry–Peach Yogurt Smoothie, 132
Ratatouille with Beans, 49
Recipe makeovers, 190
Red Clam Chowder, 70
Red peppers. See Peppers
Red snapper

in Provençal Fish, 6
Refrigerated foods to keep on hand, 189
Riboflavin, 93
Rice
   basmati, 119
   Basmati Rice and Chickpea Pilaf, 119
   Brown Rice Pilaf, 118
   Fig, Ginger, and Butternut Squash
      Risotto, 52
   Portobellos Stuffed with Spinach, Brown
      Rice, and Feta, 21
   Shrimp and Asparagus Risotto, 11
   in Tomato–Fennel Tofu Bake, 18
Risotto
   Fig, Ginger, and Butternut Squash
      Risotto, 52
   Shrimp and Asparagus Risotto, 11
Roast Beef Roll-Up, 97
Roasted Brussels Sprouts, 126
Roasted Potatoes and Baby Carrots, 124
Roasted Root Vegetable Soup, 73
Rosemary
   Quinoa and Corn Salad with Rosemary, 93
   Rosemary Popcorn, 153

S

Salads
   Arugula and Parmigiano–Reggiano Salad,
      109
   Asian Beef Salad, 83
   Beet, Orange, and Arugula Salad, 96
   Black Bean and Corn Salad, 115
   Carrot–Raisin–Apple Salad, 103
   Chunky Vegetable Salad, 102
   Crab Salad with Grapefruit, Avocado, and
      Baby Greens, 76
   Curried Chicken Salad, 79
   Greens and Herb Salad, 112
   Mediterranean Chicken Salad, 81
   Quinoa and Corn Salad with Rosemary, 93
   Shrimp, Watermelon, and Avocado
      Salad, 91
   Spicy Soba Salad, 80
   Spinach, Portobello, and Roasted Red
      Pepper Salad, 95
   Tabbouleh Salad, 111
   Tomatoes Stuffed with Shrimp Salad, 84
   Tuna–Bean Salad, 85
   Wheat Berry Salad with Almonds and

Dried Cherries, 98
Salmon
   Ginger-Poached Salmon with Orange and
      Honey, 15
   Microwave Thai Red Curry Salmon, 14
   nutrients in, 50
   Poached Salmon with Mango Salsa, 40
   Salmon in Asian Broth, 50
   Savory Salmon and Leek Packets, 47
   Wasabi Salmon Burgers, 5
Salsa(s)
   Fresh Tomato Salsa, 163
   mango, 40
   pineapple, 4
   Tomatillo Salsa, 164
Salt
   Kosher, 106
   sea, 106
Sandwiches. See also Burgers; Tacos
   Barbecue Chicken Quesadilla, 75
   Greek Chicken and Tzatziki Pitas, 87
   Quesadilla with Beans, Corn, and Green
      Chiles, 94
   Roast Beef Roll-Up, 97
   Tuna Melt, 74
   Turkey Roll-Up, 92
Sausage
   Andouille, 9
   Southern Shrimp and Sausage, 9
Sautéed Green Beans and Grape Tomatoes,
   117
Sautéed Spinach with Garlic, 125
Savory Salmon and Leek Packets, 47
Seafood
   cod, 6, 13, 60
   Crab Salad with Grapefruit, Avocado, and
      Baby Greens, 76
   Ginger-Poached Salmon with Orange and
      Honey, 15
   Green Curry Shrimp, 24
   Grilled Baja–Style Fish Tacos, 13
   halibut, 6, 13
   Mediterranean Tuna Pâté, 159
   Microwave Thai Red Curry Salmon, 14
   mussels, 16, 60
   Mussels with Fennel, Leek, and Grape
      Tomatoes, 16
   Poached Salmon with Mango Salsa, 40
   Provençal Fish, 6

red snapper, 6
salmon, 5, 14, 15, 40, 47, 50
Salmon in Asian Broth, 50
Savory Salmon and Leek Packets, 47
Seafood Stew, 60
shrimp, 11, 24, 48, 60, 84, 91
Shrimp and Asparagus Risotto, 11
Shrimp, Bean, and Feta Bake, 48
*Shrimp, Watermelon, and Avocado
Salad*, 91
Skillet Tilapia with Sautéed Spinach, 45
*Steamed Pesto-Rolled Tilapia with
Vegetables*, 29
swordfish, 13
tilapia, 29, 45, 60
Tomatoes Stuffed with Shrimp Salad, 84
tuna, 74, 85, 159
Tuna–Bean Salad, 85
Tuna Melt, 74
Wasabi Salmon Burgers, 5
Shiitake mushrooms. *See* Mushrooms
Shrimp
Green Curry Shrimp, 24
in *Seafood Stew*, 60
Shrimp and Asparagus Risotto, 11
Shrimp, Bean, and Feta Bake, 48
*Shrimp, Watermelon, and Avocado
Salad*, 91
Tomatoes Stuffed with Shrimp Salad, 84
Skillet Tilapia with Sautéed Spinach, 45
Smoothies
*Blueberry–Peach–Pomegranate
Smoothie*, 149
Raspberry–Peach Yogurt Smoothie, 132
Strawberry–Banana Smoothie, 135
Soba
Spicy Soba Salad, 80
Soups, 62–73. *See also* Stews; Chili
*Aromatic Butternut Squash and Apple
Soup*, 65
Black Bean Soup with Cilantro Cream, 66
Chicken and White Bean Soup, 69
Lentil–Vegetable Soup, 72
Mushroom–Barley Soup, 71
Red Clam Chowder, 70
Roasted Root Vegetable Soup, 73
Southwest Chicken Tortilla Soup, 64
Super Veggie Soup, 67
Southern Shrimp and Sausage, 9

Southwest Chicken Tortilla Soup, 64
Southwestern Bean Burgers, 88
Soy, nutritional value, 10
Spicy Soba Salad, 80
Spinach
in *Baked Eggs Florentine*, 140
*Portobellos Stuffed with Spinach, Brown
Rice, and Feta*, 21
in *Salmon in Asian Broth*, 50
Sautéed Spinach with Garlic, 125
Skillet Tilapia with Sautéed Spinach, 45
*Spinach, Portobello, and Roasted Red
Pepper Salad*, 95
in *Stuffed Greek Chicken Breasts*, 58
Squash, butternut
*Aromatic Butternut Squash and Apple
Soup*, 65
Black Bean and Butternut Squash Chili,
43
*Fig, Ginger, and Butternut Squash
Risotto*, 52
*Steamed Pesto-Rolled Tilapia with
Vegetables*, 29
Stews. *See also* Soups; Chili
Chicken and Barley Stew, 33
Seafood Stew, 60
Stir-fry(ies)
Chicken and Broccoli Stir-Fry, 37
*Stir-Fried Pork, Green Beans, and Shiitake
Mushrooms*, 57
Tofu Stir-Fry with Peanut Sauce, 10
Strawberry(ies)
in *Brown Sugar Yogurt Parfait*, 131
Chocolate-Covered Strawberries, 187
in *Homemade Berry Frozen Yogurt*, 183
in *Mock Berry Crème Brûlée*, 174
Strawberries with Balsamic Glaze, 181
Strawberry–Banana Smoothie, 135
Stuffed Greek Chicken Breasts, 58
Super Veggie Soup, 67
Sweet potato(es)
nutrients in, 106
Sweet Potato Fries, 106
Whipped Cider Sweet Potatoes, 113
Swordfish, 13

T
Tabbouleh Salad, 111
Tacos. *See also* Sandwiches

Eggs-Traordinary Taco, 78
Grilled Baja–Style Fish Tacos, 13
Tasty Turkey Tacos, 23
Tahini, 80
Tandoori-Style Chicken, 19
Tilapia
in *Seafood Stew*, 60
Skillet Tilapia with Sautéed Spinach, 45
*Steamed Pesto-Rolled Tilapia with
Vegetables*, 29
Toasting nuts, 21, 93
Tofu
Tofu Stir-Fry with Peanut Sauce, 10
Tomato–Fennel Tofu Bake, 18
Tomatillo Salsa, 164
Tomato(es)
Fettuccine with Tomato–Herb Sauce, 56
Fresh Tomato Salsa, 163
Lamb Burgers with Tomato–Olive Relish,
89
*Sautéed Green Beans and Grape
Tomatoes*, 117
Tomato and Basil Frittata, 139
Tomatoes Stuffed with Shrimp Salad, 84
Tomato–Fennel Tofu Bake, 18
Tortilla(s). *See also* Quesadillas; Tacos
corn, 23
Homemade Baked Tortilla Chips, 162
Pepperoni Tortilla Pizza, 155
Southwest Chicken Tortilla Soup, 64
Veggie Tortilla Pizza, 157
Tuna
Mediterranean Tuna Pâté, 159
Tuna–Bean Salad, 85
Tuna Melt, 74
Turkey
ground, types of, 46
in *Mini Meatloaves*, 46
in *Olé Pasta Casserole*, 22
Oven-Roasted Herbed Turkey Breast, 7
removing skin of, 7
Tasty Turkey Tacos, 23
Turkey Burgers with Cranberry Chutney, 86
Turkey Roll-Up, 92
Two-Bite Brownies, 171

V
Veggie Tortilla Pizza, 157
Vitamin A, 49, 56, 57, 103

Vitamin C, 3, 6, 40, 49, 56, 57, 76, 184
Vitamin K, 3, 56

W

Waffle(s)
  Whole Grain Gingerbread Waffles, 134
Wasabi Salmon Burgers, 5
Water chestnuts
  nutrients in, 37
Watermelon
  *Shrimp, Watermelon, and Avocado
    Salad*, 91
*Wheat Berry Salad with Almonds and
  Dried Cherries*, 98

Whipped Cider Sweet Potatoes, 113
White kidney beans. *See* Beans
Whole Grain Gingerbread Waffles, 134
*Whole Wheat Penne with Roasted Vegetable
  Sauce*, 36

Y

Yogurt
  in *Blueberry–Peach–Pomegranate
    Smoothie*, 149
  Brown Sugar Yogurt Parfait, 131
  Fruit Skewers with Yogurt Dipping Sauce,
    160
  Homemade Berry Frozen Yogurt, 183

with live and active cultures, 131
marinade, 19
in *Mock Berry Crème Brûlée*, 174
Raspberry–Peach Yogurt Smoothie, 132
in *Strawberry–Banana Smoothie*, 135
in tzatziki sauce, 87

Z

Zinc, 16, 37

OTHER BOOKS PUBLISHED BY
THE AMERICAN CANCER SOCIETY

Available everywhere books are sold and online at www.cancer.org/bookstore

Product Code	Title

Tools for the Health Conscious

940301	ACS's Healthy Eating Cookbook, 3rd Edition
943700	Celebrate! (Healthy Entertaining for Any Occasion)
947100	Good for You! (Reducing Your Risk of Developing Cancer)
951100	Kicking Butts (Quit Smoking and Take Charge of Your Health)
202727	National Health Education Standards: Achieving Excellence, 2nd Edition

Praise for **American Cancer Society's Healthy Eating Cookbook:**

"The *American Cancer Society's Healthy Eating Cookbook* is an important, popular, and enthusiastically recommended addition to any personal or community library's kitchen cookbook collection." —*Midwest Book Review*

Healthy Books for Children

910000	Healthy Me (A Read-Along Coloring & Activity Book)
940100	Kids' First Cookbook (Delicious-Nutritious Treats to Make Yourself!)

Praise for **Kids' First Cookbook:**

"A cookbook with a contemporary look filled with nutrition information. The uncluttered…layout is pleasing and employs colored type, drawings, and helpful photographs. A solid effort that will encourage healthy eating habits." —*School Library Journal*

Inspirational Survivor Stories

951000	Angels & Monsters (A Child's Eye View of Cancer)
946300	Crossing Divides (A Couple's Story of Cancer, Hope and Hiking Montana's Continental Divide)
954000	I Can Survive (For the Survivor in Each of Us!)

Praise for **Angels & Monsters:**

"Stunningly beautiful and thought-provoking…. Sensitive, insightful, unique, and thoroughly "kid-friendly." Highly recommended." —*Midwest Book Review*

CONTINUED

Cancer Information

963200	Cancer: What Causes It, What Doesn't
950500	Coming to Terms with Cancer (A Glossary of Cancer-Related Terms)
944902	Informed Decisions, 2nd Edition
967300	The Cancer Atlas (Chinese)
967000	The Cancer Atlas (English)
967200	The Cancer Atlas (French)
967100	The Cancer Atlas (Spanish)
967700	The Tobacco Atlas, 2nd Edition (Chinese)
967400	The Tobacco Atlas, 2nd Edition (English)
967600	The Tobacco Atlas, 2nd Edition (French)
967500	The Tobacco Atlas, 2nd Edition (Spanish)

Information for People with Cancer (Site-Specific)

953800	A Breast Cancer Journey, 2nd Edition
965800	ACS's Complete Guide to Colorectal Cancer
965200	ACS's Complete Guide to Prostate Cancer
966100	QuickFACTS™ Colon Cancer
966300	QuickFACTS™ Lung Cancer
966000	QuickFACTS™ Prostate Cancer

Symptom Management

963700	ACS's Guide to Pain Control, Revised Edition
963300	Eating Well, Staying Well During and After Cancer
965701	Lymphedema: Understanding and Managing Lymphedema After Cancer Treatment

Support for Families and Caregivers

943500	Cancer in the Family (Helping Children Cope with a Parent's Illness)
466000	Cancer Support Groups (A Guide for Facilitators)
952700	Caregiving (A Step-by-Step Resource for Caring for the Person with Cancer at Home, Revised Edition)
951200	Couples Confronting Cancer (Keeping Your Relationship Strong)
965100	When the Focus Is on Care (Palliative Care and Cancer)

Support for Children

951300	Because…Someone I Love Has Cancer (Kids' Activity Book)
968000	Mom and the Polka-Dot Boo-Boo
949600	Our Mom Has Cancer (hard cover)
945700	Our Mom Has Cancer (paperback)
968200	Our Dad Is Getting Better
968100	Our Mom Is Getting Better